KT-485-660

HOW TO GO VEGAN

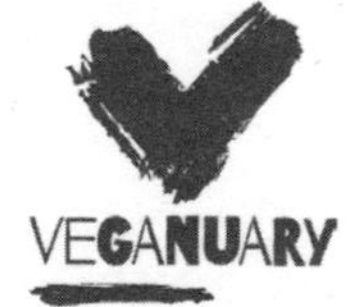

HOW TO GO VEGAN

The why, the how, and everything you need to make going vegan easy

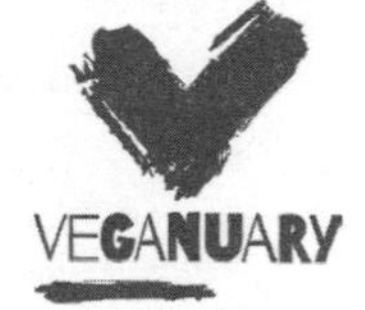

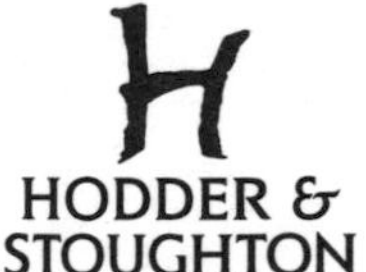

First published in Great Britain in 2017 by Hodder & Stoughton
An Hachette UK company

3

Author Kate Schuler 2017

A CIP catalogue record for this title is available from the British Library

Hardback ISBN 9781473680968
eBook ISBN 9781473680975

Typeset in Celeste 11/15.5 pt by
Palimpsest Book Production Limited, Falkirk, Stirlingshire

Printed and bound in the UK by Clays Ltd, St Ives plc

Hodder & Stoughton policy is to use papers that are natural, renewable and recyclable products and made from wood grown in sustainable forests. The logging and manufacturing processes are expected to conform to the environmental regulations of the country of origin.

No animal products were used in the manufacture of this book.

Hodder & Stoughton Ltd
Carmelite House
50 Victoria Embankment
London EC4Y 0DZ

www.hodder.co.uk

CONTENTS

FOREWORD

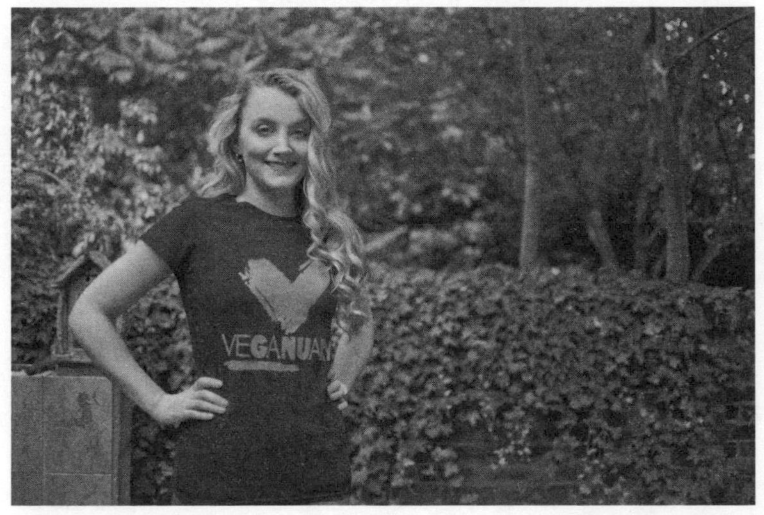

Evanna Lynch, *actress and vegan activist*

Whether you are already vegan, vegetarian, pescatarian, flexitarian, v-curious or you're just contemplating making changes to your diet, then you've already made one huge leap on your journey – you're reading this book! Simply by setting the intention to learn about living a cruelty-free life I believe you are vegan at heart, which is the first bold step to being vegan in practice.

In a way veganism is not such a radical change; it can be more like a return to self and simply aligning your practices with your principles. Most of us are not brought up or socially conditioned to choose the vegan option, and yet most of us would agree we want to live a life that doesn't cause unnecessary suffering to other living beings. Going vegan, I felt like I was becoming more myself and very quickly felt more comfortable in my skin. It's exciting to uncover another piece of your identity, liberating in fact. Veganism was a big piece of the puzzle for me, and it might be for you too.

But while recognising that I was against animal cruelty in any form was one thing, actually becoming vegan took some time, patience, research and, most of all, community with other vegans. I read *Eating Animals* by Jonathan Safran Foer and felt thoroughly well-versed in the reasons why I was now vegan, and riled up to revamp my whole life. But I forgot to account for the fact that I was unlearning two decades' worth of living a completely different lifestyle, and that there was a method to making going vegan easier. I quickly learned that going vegan required compassion for myself as much as for the animals and I urge you to be gentle with yourself as you work towards integrating veganism seamlessly into your life. I wish I could have followed up *Eating Animals* with this beautiful, inspiring, information-packed tome you're reading, which feels like a friendly vegan fairy godmother taking your hand and guiding you down your personal tailor-made path to becoming the best vegan you can be. *How to Go Vegan* is a fantastic introduction to all of the reasons why you might want to give veganism a go, how you can live it, and will be something you can go back to again and again and share with your sceptical mother and curious cousin alike.

One thing I'd like to imprint on your brain is that veganism is not about being perfect. And it isn't about rules and restrictions; it is about living with compassion and mindfulness – for animals, for yourself, for other humans, for our planet. You will struggle, you may make mistakes, you might feel like you're being awkward, but you'll learn that there's no such thing as a perfect vegan. You may even be tentative about sharing your new vegan life or using the V word at all because you're afraid of facing judgement, as I was. But once you do 'come out' as vegan you'll find that the vegan community is incredibly loving and supportive, friendly and thoughtful, and they make the sassiest memes. You'll find that people are just pleased that you want to help save animals' lives and the planet, and they're eager to help you on your journey. So talk to people and find your mentors and role models in the community – your vibe attracts your tribe, as they say! Most of all, just focus on doing your personal best from day to day.

The best piece of advice I got as a new vegan was to introduce delicious new vegan foods to my diet before cutting things out – to make my vegan life feel joyful and abundant – and I believe that is the way to make it sustainable. So start to try different plant milks and meat replacements alongside what you would normally eat, until they become your everyday norm, and the meat, eggs and dairy can fall out of your life without leaving a huge hungry hole behind. If you immerse yourself in all these new delicious vegan foods (and make a point to treat yo'self often) then it won't feel like you are depriving yourself of anything – instead you've opened up a whole new world of options. Yes, it will be an adjustment and you may find yourself causing a traffic jam in the vegetable aisle of your grocery store googling the difference between a yam and a sweet potato (helpful tip: nobody really knows the difference but they are closely related cousins in the root vegetable family) but you've got this, and you've also got the benefit of the collective wisdom and experience of the Veganuary team right here in front of you, and believe me, they know what they're talking about.

And when you hear people saying that vegans are 'extreme' and it's a lifestyle of sacrifice remember that the opposite is in fact true – it's about celebrating food and life! It really is a beautiful lifestyle and I trust when you fully dive in you will fall in love with it, as I have. This book is a great first step. I think you'll find that it helps to demystify veganism and show you that it's not that complicated after all. Veganuary are doing amazing work helping people give veganism a try for a month, and whatever your goals are, I think you'll find that you are happier, healthier and more content with yourself than ever before.

With lots of love and good vibes to you as you embark on your vegan journey!

Evanna xox

INTRODUCTION

You've bought this book – or been given it – because you're the kind of person who cares about something. It might be animal welfare, the environment or world hunger. It could be water shortages, land degradation or deforestation. Or perhaps your concerns relate to climate change, loss of wildlife, antibiotic resistance, pollution or looking after your own health. If you care about any of these things – *and who doesn't?* – then it's natural you would want to do your bit, to make choices that don't create greater suffering in the world and to protect our environment.

It's easy to feel helpless in the face of global problems. We may think we can have no impact no matter what we do, and that these issues require national governments and international partnerships to find solutions. We may think that one person, one ordinary person, can't make a difference. But we'd be wrong. There is something all of us can do that helps ease the burden on the planet, promotes well-being, protects wildlife and aids the world's poorest, and we can do it three times a day. Every day. It is, of course, our food choices.

What we choose to buy, cook and eat has consequences that extend way beyond our taste buds and bellies. The breakfast bacon may have come from a factory-farmed pig whose feed was grown on land where ancient rainforests once stood, who was fed antibiotics routinely just to keep him alive and whose meat, when processed, is known to cause bowel cancer in people. Or what about the milk in our tea? It may have come from a cow who lived her whole life in a shed, who was fed grain that could have instead been used to feed the world's most hungry and whose slurry contributes significantly to climate change. We're not told these things on the label but it doesn't make them any less true.

As the full impact of animal agriculture on our world becomes clearer, more and more people are choosing to avoid eating animal products altogether. They may call themselves 'vegan' or 'plant-based', or they may not choose a label at all, but the number of people who avoid meat, milk and eggs is rising exponentially, and this is happening all around the world.

In the United States six per cent of the population now identify as vegan[1]. In the United Kingdom, there has been a 260 per cent rise over the past decade, with now more than half a million vegans in the country[2].

The range of vegan foods available has skyrocketed to

meet this booming market. In the US, vegan product launches grew by a third in one year,[3] while in the UK, the biggest supermarket chain Tesco says that demand for vegetarian and vegan ready-meals and snacks has soared by 40 per cent in one year.[4] And Australia – the third fastest-growing vegan market in the world after the United Arab Emirates and China – expects to see sales grow by more than 60 per cent by 2020.[5]

All this delicious, readily available food makes it even easier for people to choose animal-free products, and this helps create more vegans, who then demand more delicious vegan products, and that creates even more vegans. You see the pattern. This is a movement with powerful momentum behind it. In fact, it appears to be unstoppable.

Perhaps you're already vegan, vegetarian or v-curious, or you've tried being vegan and fallen off the wagon. Maybe you have friends and family who are vegan or interested in giving it a go. This book is for you. We don't ask for perfection, or for you to make yourself miserable by putting too much pressure on yourself. It's OK to make mistakes and have the odd slip-up. Most vegans did exactly the same when they started out, too.

WHAT EXACTLY *IS* A VEGAN?

Vegans eat no animal products at all, from the obvious items like meat, milk and eggs to the less obvious like honey. This book focuses on the foods that we eat, but most vegans will also avoid wearing animal products like fur, leather, silk and wool, and will also choose household products and cosmetics that contain no animal-derived ingredients.

We hope this book, which is intended as a practical guide to introduce you to plant-based eating, will help you on your way. Read it from cover to cover or just dip in as you wish. In it, we explain not just *why* we should embrace a plant-based diet – for animals, health and the environment – but *how* that can be done. We take the mystery out of where to shop, what to buy and how to keep eating the foods you love. We discuss nutrition and pass on our top tips for making sure you get everything you need from the foods you eat. We reveal the animal ingredients that can sneak into the foods you buy, and give you some great meal plans to get you started. We give you the support you need to try vegan for a month, from getting started on Day 1 to what you might decide to do on Day 32. And we talk you through how to deal with questions from family and friends, advise on how to travel as a vegan and offer our top choices for further reading and viewing.

WHAT IS VEGANUARY?

Veganuary is a UK charity with global reach that encourages people around the world to try vegan for a month in January or throughout the year, alongside tens of thousands of others. We offer support and advice and a non-judgemental approach for everyone who registers to take part at veganuary.com.

'For me it took 38 years to be ready to make that full commitment, and some people may never get to that stage, but Veganuary is a great opportunity to try it out. I genuinely think that for a lot of people, it will be much easier than they would have anticipated. They'll feel different, they'll have more energy and they'll just feel cleaner.'

Jasmine Harman, television presenter, UK, Veganuary Class of 2014

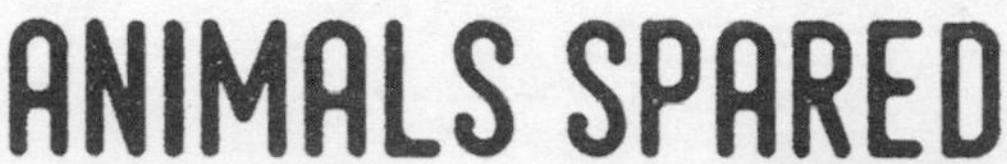

14,012,825

ANIMALS WERE SPARED AS A RESULT OF VEGANUARY 2017

To understand how we calculated lives spared please visit:
https://veganuary.com/blog/did-veganuary-2017-help-animals/

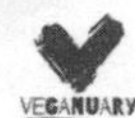

IMPROVED HEALTH

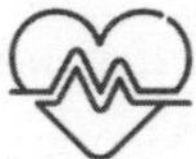

97% FEEL HEALTHIER

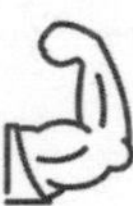

87% HAVE MORE ENERGY

87% LOST WEIGHT

The survey results from Veganuary's #Classof2017 suggest most people see an improvement in their health after just one month.

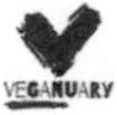

WHY TRY VEGAN?

• • •

While this book is all about the *how*, we need to begin by talking about the *why*. These are the reasons that most people give for trying vegan in the first place, and they are also what motivates them to stick with it in the face of difficult questions, mocking friends or a poor food offering when eating out.

And there are lots of reasons why people try vegan for 31 days – animals, the environment, sustainability, world hunger, personal health, global human health or just because it's a new challenge.

Whatever the reason that prompts someone to try plant-based eating in the first place, it often becomes just one of many good reasons why they choose to stick with it in the long term. For example, someone may try vegan to see how it boosts their athletic performance but along the way find out how chickens are factory-farmed; so this becomes another motivating factor. Another person may cut out animal products because they learn that calves are killed by the dairy industry but they stay vegan because they find out more about that industry's contribution to climate change. Everyone is different, and all reasons are equally valid.

> 'This was just the right path for me. I felt like as soon as I went vegan, I was more myself, like I was just living according to what I believed, which is such a freeing thing once you finally commit to it.'
>
> *Evanna Lynch, actor, UK*

But the top reason people give – the reason that most people say motivated them to try vegan – is to end animal suffering.

> 'Going vegan is the best thing I could have done, for animals, the planet and my own health. I only wish I'd done it sooner.'
>
> *Miranda W., Surrey, UK, Veganuary Class of 2017*

WHY TRY VEGAN –
YOUR TWO-MINUTE GUIDE

If you're short of time and keen to get to the how as quickly as possible, this is your two-minute guide to all the reasons why people try vegan. Once you've read it, you may want to jump straight into the practical tips and get started. That's fine. Go right ahead and turn to page 61 – or you may prefer to read a little more about any or all of the reasons. It's your call. Whatever you choose, you might like to revisit this 'why' section later on to refresh your knowledge or if you feel your motivation flagging.

REASONS FOR TAKING PART

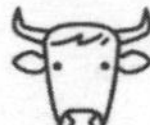 47% FOR ANIMALS

 32% FOR HEALTH

 13% FOR ENVIRONMENT

8% FOR OTHER REASONS

People take part in Veganuary for a number of reasons. A concern for animals is always the most common one, but increasingly participants are concerned about their health and the environment too.

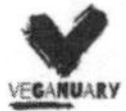

ANIMALS

This is the top reason why people go vegan. It's obvious that animals must die for people to eat meat, but most people are shocked to learn that animals are killed in the egg and dairy industries, too. Male calves are often unwanted by-products of the dairy industry, and billions of day-old chicks are killed because they are the wrong sex to lay eggs. Did you know that most chickens and pigs are still intensively farmed, and that there are no welfare laws governing the slaughter of fish at sea?

'This decision has really made me consider everything I put in my body and how to honour myself and treat myself well. I never really felt connected to animals but now that I don't eat them, I feel more love in my heart for all beings. You can do almost anything for a month! Do it not only as a kindness to yourself, but as a kindness to all living beings and the planet we inhabit.'

Bekah D., New York, USA

ENVIRONMENT

Eating animal products is one of the top four ways each of us contributes to climate-changing emissions, along with driving cars, flying and having children. The great news is that we can help protect the planet with every plant-based meal we eat. Since producing vegan foods also requires less land and water than producing animal products, being vegan is also great news for forests, hedgerows, waterways and all the world's other wild places and their inhabitants.

WORLD HUNGER

What we choose to eat has an impact on people all over the world. Currently, we produce more than enough food for everyone on the planet, but still one billion people go hungry every day. War, poverty and natural disasters all play a part, but so too does the fact that we feed one-third of the world's cereal harvest and 90 per cent of the world's soya harvest to farmed animals instead of to people.[1]

PERSONAL HEALTH

People often report that their skin, hair, sinuses, digestion and sleep improve after eating vegan foods for 31 days. Others say they have more energy, better mental clarity and their sporting performance improves. Some have told us that their chronic fatigue symptoms have reduced and that their depression symptoms were relieved. In the long term, eating a plant-based diet can also reduce the risk of high blood pressure, heart disease, type 2 diabetes and some cancers. Great news all round!

'Veganism has changed my life in so many ways. It changed the way I physically feel. I didn't realise how tired and bloated I felt all the time until I stopped eating meat. My skin is clear and smoother, my digestion has improved and my anxiety has significantly decreased.'

Julie M., Arizona, USA, Veganuary Class of 2017

GLOBAL HEALTH

Farming animals has the potential to affect huge swathes of the global population. Many of the diseases that harm and kill people started out in farmed animals, and new diseases and strains are still emerging. Avian flu is just one example of an animal-borne disease that continues to kill people. The vast amounts of antibiotics we use to keep farmed animals alive has contributed to the emergence of antibiotic-resistant superbugs, and this also threatens people worldwide.

FOR THE ADVENTURE

Some people try 31 days of vegan eating because of the challenge of trying something different. Maybe they want to experience new ways of shopping, cooking and eating because they're stuck in a culinary rut. Perhaps they feel their health needs a bit of a boost. They may not have any preconceived ideas about what being vegan will do for them, but they try it just because.

> 'Best. Decision. Ever!'
>
> *Albie J., London, UK, Veganuary Class of 2017*

Whatever your reason for trying vegan: we wish you the best of luck. This book is here to help you.

FOR ANIMALS

'It was such a good decision! I no longer feel guilty about what I eat – my diet now aligns with my beliefs that animals aren't for us to use, and that we are all equal.'

Lana M., Auckland, New Zealand, Veganuary Class of 2017

We know this section will be tough and upsetting to read. But we also know that ending animal suffering is the number one reason why people choose to go vegan. So if you're finding this section difficult, give yourself a break, move forward in the book, and come back to it later. Remember how important it is to be informed about our food choices, and re-reading this section will be a great boost for your motivation later on.

From the invasive process of artificial insemination to gassing newborn male chicks and surgery without pain relief, farmed animals suffer the world over for their meat, milk and eggs.

Most meat – including 94 per cent of the chicken sold in the UK[1] and more than 99 per cent of all farmed animals in the US[2] – comes from animals who have been intensively reared. They are kept in cages and pens, or crammed inside immense barns with tens of thousands of other animals. It is impossible for farmers to check every individual chicken, duck or turkey each day, and so the sick and injured are often simply left to die.

Some countries do have higher welfare standards than others. Switzerland, for example, has banned the cages known as 'farrowing crates' where pigs are confined to give birth. In Sweden, all pigs must have straw. These, though, are exceptions. In most other countries – including the UK, Canada, USA and Australia – many egg-laying hens are still farmed in cages, mother pigs can be kept in crates for prolonged periods and straw for bedding and rooting is often denied.

It's easy to forget that every one of the billions of farmed animals in the world is an individual who forms friendship bonds, has preferences and displays a distinct character. To truly understand this, we'd recommend a visit to your nearest farmed-animal sanctuary to meet the rescued dairy cows, pigs and chickens. Not only is this one of the most uplifting experiences you will ever have, it also removes all doubt about there being two different kinds of animals: those we share our homes with, and others that we eat. At sanctuaries like The Retreat (UK), Edgar's Mission (Australia) and Catskill Animal Sanctuary and Animal Place (both in the US), this distinction breaks down, and you will see that the sheep in the field isn't really so different from the dog on your sofa. Both like a belly rub, and will steal your sandwiches when you're not looking!

Deep down, many of us may have an uneasy feeling that there is something not quite right with eating meat, but we try to take some comfort in the notion that farmed animals have a good life and a humane death. We're sorry. This just isn't the case. Difficult as this section on animals is to read, we urge you to give it a try. After all, the suffering of animals is the leading reason why people choose to become vegan. And we promise that things will lighten up again in the next section!

Take a deep breath. Ready?

CHICKENS

Anyone who's ever met a chicken will know what huge characters they can be. They are active, inquisitive and love to root around, foraging and exploring. They dust-bathe and preen to keep their skin and feathers in tip-top shape, and love to sunbathe, lying on their sides, wings outstretched, eyes closed.

For farmed chickens, whether they are reared for their meat ('broilers') or for their eggs, none of this is possible.

Almost all broiler chickens are kept inside huge warehouse-style hangars with tens of thousands of other birds. Because they have been bred to grow as big as possible as quickly as possible, their bodies outgrow their bone strength and their legs may break beneath them. Those who cannot stand up suffer skin burns from the ammonia in the litter that covers the floor. Their hearts cannot cope with their ballooning weight, and heart failure is all too common. The dead may be taken away, or just left to rot among the living birds.

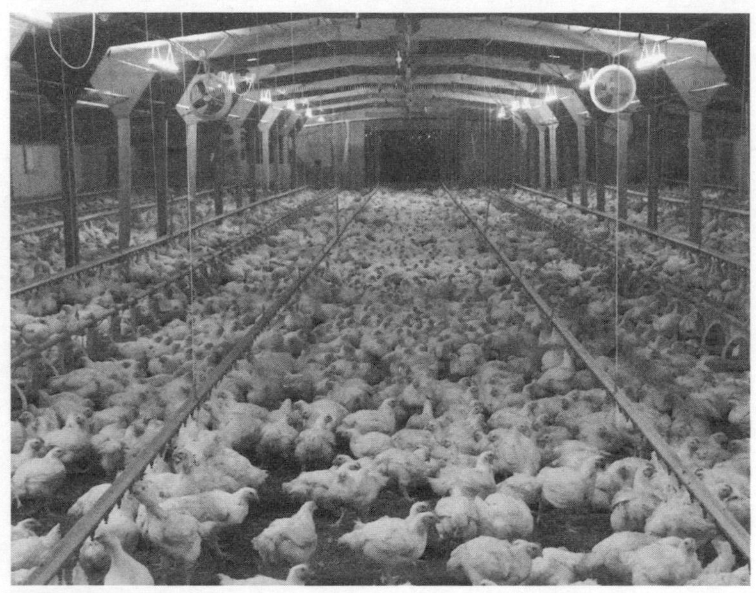

A free range chicken farm.

Egg-laying hens scarcely get a better time of it. Most spend their whole reproductive lives in cages, even across the European Union where battery cages were banned in 2012. When that law was brought in, the industry could have moved to free range systems, but instead it simply lobbied for bigger cages. And it won. The new 'improved' colony cages have a perch and a scratch pad and are big enough to house 80 birds – but they are still cages. Where the original battery cages allowed each hen space the size of an A4 sheet of paper (which is just a little larger than letter-sized paper in Canada and the US), the additional space in the colony cages is less than the size of one beer mat per hen.[3]

In the US, 85 per cent of eggs come from caged hens[4] and in Australia, more than half of the country's egg-laying flock are caged.[5] None of these billions of birds are able to express their natural behaviours, such as nesting, foraging and dust-bathing. Artificial lights are switched on for prolonged periods to encourage them to lay even more eggs. A lot of calcium is required to make all those eggshells, and the mineral is taken from the birds' bones, which leaves them susceptible to broken legs and wings. It's a price the industry is willing to pay for plentiful eggs.

These birds might naturally have lived ten years or more, but by the age of 18 months they are past their productive peak, and there is no happy retirement. They are loaded into crates and shipped to slaughterhouses, where they are killed and their scrawny, broken-down bodies turned into processed products such as pies, soups and nuggets. Poultry is specifically excluded from the Humane Methods of Slaughter Act in the US, so there are no laws to protect them from suffering at slaughter.[6]

The hens themselves are not the only victims of the egg industry. With such a high turnover of birds, the industry must continually breed more. Half of the eggs that hatch are, inevitably, male. They're the wrong sex to lay eggs, and the wrong breed for meat, and so millions of male chicks are killed on their very first day of life. In the UK, they're gassed to death. In Australia and the US, they may instead be fed alive into mincing machines. This same fate awaits male chicks hatched on free range and organic farms. For more information on 'higher welfare' farming, see page 120.

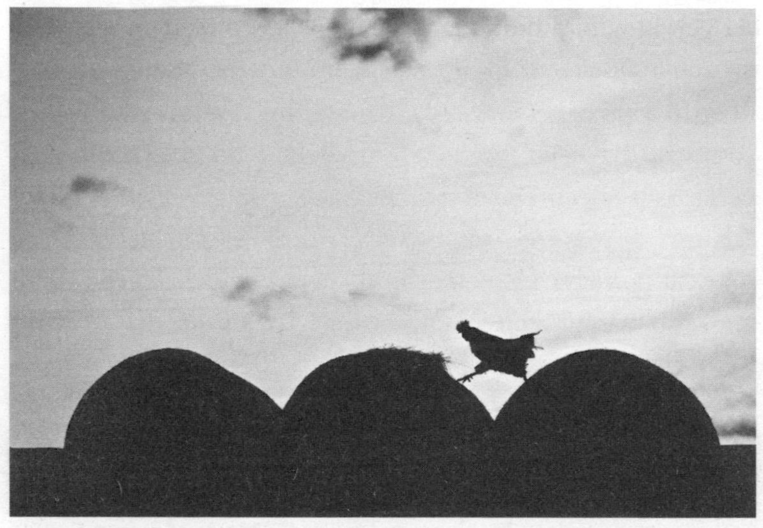

A cockerel free at the Retreat Animal Rescue Farm Sanctuary in the UK.

COWS

Cows possess many of the same emotional qualities as people. Like us, some are playful, cheeky and outgoing, while others are more sensitive, thoughtful or shy. All are capable of happiness, though, and cows literally jump for joy when given reason to. But cows reared for their milk and those reared for their meat suffer physically and emotionally.

Like all female mammals, dairy cows must be made pregnant to produce milk. This is usually done via artificial insemination, with one hand in the cow's anus to manipulate her cervix while the other inserts a straw of semen into her vagina. Suddenly, milk doesn't seem quite so natural!

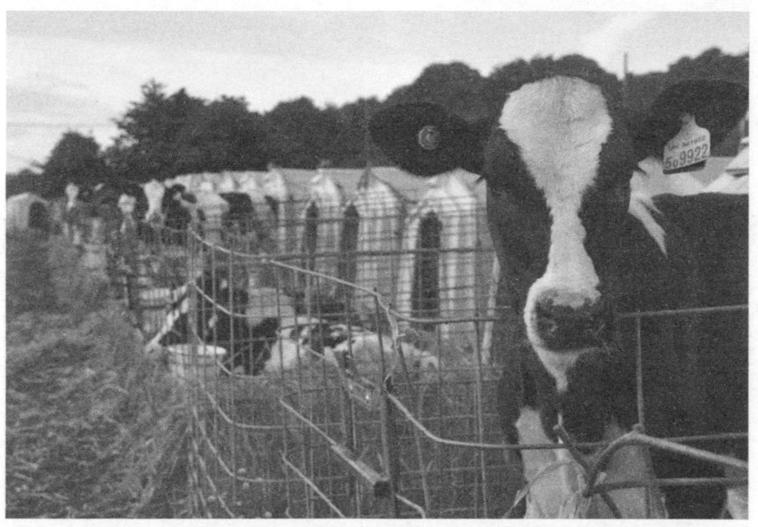

Calves are taken from their mothers in the dairy industry.

The milk she produces is intended for her calf but instead of suckling for a year, calves are taken away from their mums within hours of birth to stop them drinking all that valuable milk. Male calves are often deemed worthless and may be shot at birth, while some are reared as veal or trucked straight to the slaughterhouse.[7] Females, who will go on to become 'milkers' themselves, may be moved to hutches where, instead of receiving the comfort, warmth and security that newborns need from their mothers, they are kept confined and alone.

The separation is traumatic for both mother and calf. They call for one another, sometimes for days, with some mothers pacing back and forth, searching for a way to be reunited with their lost young. A dairy cow will lose calf after calf as she is repeatedly impregnated and near-continuously milked, and pushed to her biological limits. When her milk production declines, she is worn out – or 'spent' as the industry calls it – and will be sent to slaughter. She could have lived to 15 or 20 years old, but will be killed at just five or six, and her body made into low-grade meat products. Even heavily pregnant dairy cows are slaughtered[8, 9, 10, 11] – because of illness or age, or because the farmer did not know they were pregnant[12] – with some calves being born and dying on the slaughterhouse floor.

In some areas of the world, like New Zealand, dairy cows can live outdoors all year round because the climate allows it.[13] In other parts of the world, dairy cows are turned out to graze for around six months of the year, and the rest of the time they stand around in a barn. An increasing number of dairy cows are never allowed outside at all. They are intensively farmed. After all, why waste valuable time getting cows in from fields when you could just keep them in and bring food to them? This is called 'zero-grazing' and is exactly what it sounds like: the cows never graze. Permanently housing cows inside can lead to two common causes of suffering: mastitis, which is a painful infection of their udders, and lameness, meaning they will struggle to walk, usually due to crippling pain.

Life is no picnic for cows reared for their meat either. Calves may be dehorned, castrated and branded, often all at once. All of these legally permitted mutilations may be performed without anaesthetic[14] and, in most countries, no pain relief is required by law.

Whether they are 'grass-raised' or kept in intensive systems where they never see the outdoors, their lives are over when they reach the required weight. They are just 18 months old;[15] naturally, they could have lived for twenty years or more.

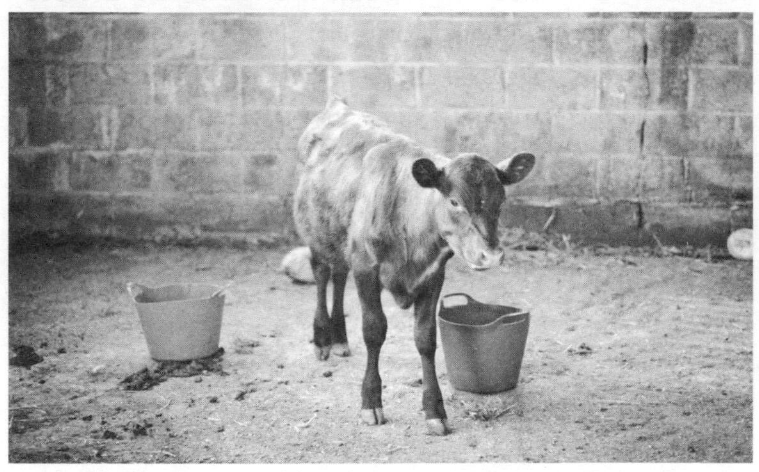

A rescued calf at the Retreat Animal Rescue Farm Sanctuary in the UK.

PIGS

Pigs are every bit as intelligent, fun-loving and charismatic as dogs. Yet pigs are reared on intensive farms in a way that would horrify us – and lead to animal cruelty charges – if it was done to our canine pal Fido.

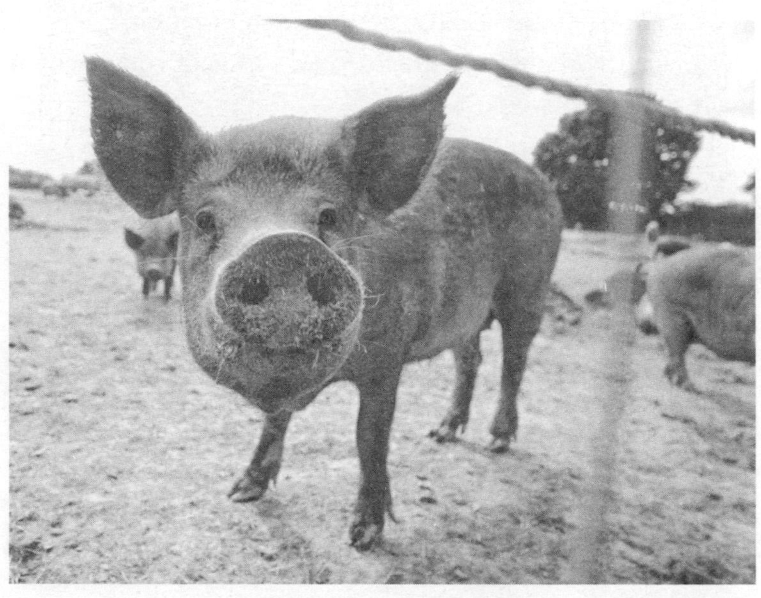

A rescued pig at the Retreat Animal Rescue Farm Sanctuary in the UK

Gestation crates – metal enclosures that confine female pigs throughout each 16-week pregnancy – are banned in the UK, but are still legal in Canada, Australia and most US states.[16] Even in the countries where gestation crates are banned, farrowing crates remain legal. Female pigs may be held in these tiny pens, barely bigger than their own bodies, for several weeks while they complete their pregnancy and give birth. The crates are so small the sows cannot even turn round.

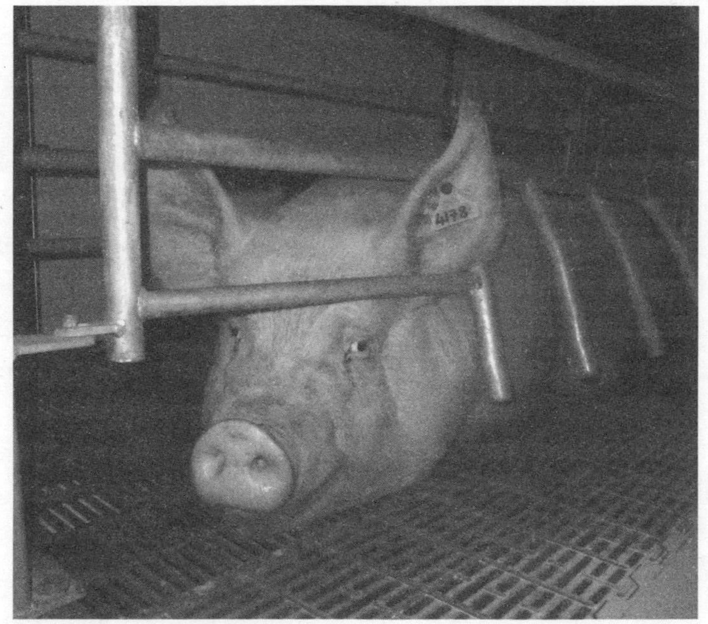

Pigs are confined to farrowing crates for weeks.

In the wild, pigs would find a private place to build a nest in which to give birth. On farms, all they have are the metal bars that prevent them moving and a concrete or metal floor that can cause painful pressure sores. In desperation, they go through the motions of nest-building, but it is, of course, totally futile.[17]

When born, the piglets are able to suckle from their mother but she is separated from them by the bars of the crate and is not able to reach them to nuzzle them. If they are sick, all she can do is watch them die. She will be kept in this confinement until the young are taken from her, then she will be returned to a pen to be impregnated again. And again, and again, until she is exhausted and her body can no longer endure the strain. Then she will be sent to slaughter as a 'cull sow', and her body turned into low-quality products like pork pies and sausages.

Pigs have been bred to have the largest litters possible, and many piglets are stillborn, or die at birth or soon after. They rarely receive veterinary care. Investigators regularly find their tiny bodies abandoned in the aisles of the units or dumped inside bin bags.

In nature, weaning is a gradual process, often taking three to four months. On farms, the separation of mother and piglets after just three to four weeks[18] causes distress to them both. As with cows and their calfs, it is quite common for them to call out to one another in the vain hope of being reunited.[19]

Soon after birth, piglets will have their tails cut off, their teeth clipped or ground down and, in many countries, they will also be castrated, all without anaesthetic. The pig industry claims that the first two procedures are necessary to prevent piglets from injuring one another. However, pigs rarely harm one another when living wild. It is a problem related to their overcrowded, stressful living conditions, where boredom is rife.

Piglets may be slaughtered from the age of two weeks to produce 'whole suckling pig', but most are killed when they are around four to six months old. Their mothers are put through between three and five pregnancies before they are also slaughtered,[20] usually at around 18 months to two years old.[21] They could have lived to the age of 20.

And all this because we choose a meat sausage over a meat-style veggie one.

SHEEP

Sheep are farmed for their meat, milk and wool. They are often misunderstood, and derided as being 'stupid' simply because they flock together for protection, in the same way that some birds and fish do. When they feel safe and secure, sheep will show that they are bright and inquisitive, loving and gentle, and often extremely cheeky. On farms, they're just not given the opportunity to be themselves.

If ewes were able to breed naturally, they would give birth in spring. Now, though, many are forced to give birth in the dead of winter so that the meat is already on the shelves by spring and can be marketed as new season lamb.[22] In Australia, every year as many as 15 million lambs die within 48 hours of birth due to exposure to cold weather and lack of shelter.[23] It's the same sad story around the world.[24, 25]

Have you ever wondered why ewes on farms all give birth

around the same time? It's not a natural cycle. It's done deliberately to ensure lambing takes place at a convenient time for the farmer, and is achieved by implanting hormones under the ewes' skin or inserting hormone sponges into their vaginas to synchronise the flock's fertility.[26]

Insemination may be done artificially, too, with the semen collected from a ram using an artificial vagina or by an electric probe inserted into the ram's anus.[27] The semen is then either introduced through the cervix while the ewe is strapped to a rack, or introduced surgically through the ewe's abdomen.[28] So far, so unnatural.

Left to nature, ewes would give birth to a single lamb. However, through human manipulation, many sheep are now selectively bred to produce two or even three lambs, which is intended to increase the industry's profitability. Since ewes have just two teats, a third lamb will be given to a different ewe, bottle-fed, or force-fed through a tube into his or her stomach.

Because it is common to see sheep in fields and on hillsides, we think their lives are rather enjoyable. But we tend not to be on those hillsides when they flood,[29] or when the heat of the summer raises the risk of the unpleasant infection fly strike,[30] or in the depths of winter when snow makes finding food impossible.[31]

On top of this, sheep suffer a host of health problems and are given an array of drugs to try to prevent or manage unpleasant conditions such as scald, foot rot, scrapie, mastitis, lameness and even blindness.

Lambs may be killed when they are between three and five months old, although some are slaughtered as young as six weeks old.[32] They might otherwise have lived for ten years or more. Their mothers will also be killed when age, lameness, udder infections or prolapse mean they are no longer profitable.[33]

FISH

It's not so easy to warm to cold-blooded animals, but research shows that fish are smart enough to use tools, can communicate and have distinct personalities, just like people do.

Commercial fishing vessels can capture tens of thousands of fish at a time, with animals becoming exhausted as they desperately try to outswim the net. When pulled to the surface, those at the bottom are crushed by the weight of fish above them. The rapid change in pressure causes their swim bladders to overinflate, and their stomachs and intestines to be pushed out through their mouths and anuses. Their eyes distort, bulge and can be pushed out of their sockets.

The animals are then dropped onto the ship's deck, where those who are still alive will suffocate – a process that can take several minutes. Others, like tuna, are hoisted from the water with a hook, and killed by a spike forced through their brains.

In fish farms, fish are packed into small, often filthy enclosures. The overcrowded conditions cause a third of them to die, and an array of chemicals is used to try to prevent even more from succumbing. In this stressful environment, many fish will bite off the fins, tails and eyes of others, a distressing and destructive behaviour seen in other factory-farmed animals.

Despite an ever-increasing number of studies that show aquatic species can feel pain, there are still no welfare laws governing the humane slaughter of fish at sea, and in most countries there are no welfare requirements for slaughter on farms, either. With little or no legal protection, some truly terrible things are done to aquatic species. Lobsters and crabs may be boiled alive, while farmed shrimps are deliberately blinded in a procedure designed to boost their fertility. 'Eyestalk ablation' happens in almost every shrimp production facility in the world.[34]

> '[Going vegan] is one of my proudest decisions and has made me feel like I'm really doing my part for animals. I feel healthier and more contented that I'm not contributing to the suffering of animals.'
>
> *Alice C., Sussex, UK, Veganuary Class of 2017*

SLAUGHTERHOUSES

The lives of most farmed animals are based on deprivation, suffering and loss. For most, there is no 'good life', and nor is there a humane death. In the US, the laws that are designed to ensure animals are slaughtered humanely specifically exempt chickens, turkeys, ducks, geese, rabbits and fish, which means that the vast majority of animals killed have no right to a humane death.

In the UK, Australia and elsewhere, campaigners have filmed inside slaughterhouses and revealed that the welfare laws that do exist are often ignored, with animals being kicked, beaten and abused to their deaths. The laws that demand animals be stunned before slaughter are often not properly adhered to, and animals may be partially stunned or not stunned at all, and still go to the knife.

But perhaps the most shocking thing seen in these under-cover investigations is the fear that animals display: the sheep running in circles, throwing themselves over and over at the walls, the doors, the gates, anywhere to try to find a way out. Some even leap through the hatch that leads to the slaughter room, and land in the blood pit below their bleeding companions.

These investigations have shown cows being shot up to four times in the head with a captive bolt-gun in an attempt to stun them. They lie on the ground, looking up at the slaughterman, blinking and waiting for the next attempt. The investigations show the pain of electrical stunning, which all too often imparts a powerful electric shock instead of rendering the animal unconscious. They've shown pigs convulsing and gasping for air as the cage they are in is lowered into a gas chamber.

In these investigations, we see the pitiless nature of this business: the ewe being stunned while her lamb is still suckling from her; the injured pigs, too lame to walk, kicked and prodded and dragged through the slaughterhouse by their ears; the animals screaming in pain on the floor while a worker stands over them, taunting them. The casual indifference to the fear and suffering of these helpless creatures is demonstrated with every kick, punch and blow inflicted. It's the nature of the business that workers must become desensitised to the animals' fear.

Animals in slaughterhouses are not euthanised like a much-loved dog or cat. There is no humane way to kill an animal who does not want to die, but slaughterhouses are particularly ruthless: the slaughter line has to keep moving; no matter how hard they might try, no animal escapes.

> ***'If slaughterhouses had glass walls, everyone would be vegetarian.'***
>
> Paul McCartney

BEES

We owe bees a lot. We rely on them – and other insect pollinators – for apples, berries, cucumbers, almonds, beans, broccoli, carrots and many more of the foods that we eat and love.[35] Bees collect pollen and nectar from the flowers of these plants, pollinating as they go. Back at the hive, the nectar's content is reduced by being passed from mouth to mouth until it becomes honey. Bees do all this to create food that will see the hive through winter, not because they are worried about what people are going to have on their toast.

Commercial bee-keepers take the honey and substitute it with a sugar-water solution, which has neither the broad range of nutrients the bees need nor the power to protect their immune systems.[36] This, coupled with exposure to pesticides (including the now-infamous neonicotinoids) and destructive varroa mites, means these insects are facing a rough future.

But that's not all. Some commercial bee-keepers kill and replace the queens to ensure that their queen is always young and fertile, and even 'cull' whole hives after harvesting the honey as it is cheaper than feeding the bees through the winter months. Of course, they wouldn't need feeding if someone hadn't taken their honey.

THANK YOU

We know that this was a tough section to get through. Reading about what animals have to endure so that people can eat their meat, milk, eggs and even the animals' own food (honey) is emotionally challenging. No matter how hard it is for us to face it, we have to remember how much harder it is for the animals to live it. And it's not just the animals we've mentioned that suffer. Most ducks, turkeys and geese are reared in factory farm sheds like chickens; rabbits are reared in cages like egg-laying hens; and goats raised for their meat and milk may be kept inside barns and never see the light of day.

It's no surprise that the way we farm and slaughter animals is the main reason people give for trying vegan, but it's not the only reason . . .

FOR THE ENVIRONMENT

A growing number of people are eating plant-based foods to help protect the environment. The connection may not be as immediately obvious as with animals – after all, it's pretty clear that eating animals harms them – but what we choose to eat has a direct and significant impact on climate change, pollution, water and land usage, as well as on wild animals and their habitats.

Prepare to be shocked!

> *'If we really want to reduce the human impact on the environment, the simplest and cheapest thing anyone can do is to eat less meat. Behind most of the joints of beef or chicken on our plates is a phenomenally wasteful, land- and energy-hungry system of farming that devastates forests, pollutes oceans, rivers, seas and air, depends on coal and oil, and is significantly responsible for climate change.'*[1]

These are the words of John Vidal, Environment Editor at the *Guardian* newspaper in the UK, and he's right – except he forgot to include the egg and dairy industries. If we really want to protect the planet, cutting down on all these products is the very least we can do.

GREENHOUSE GAS EMISSIONS

The production of meat, milk and eggs relies inherently on crude oil.[2] Every link in the chain that brings meat from farm to table demands energy: the production of fertiliser that is put on the land to grow feed; powering farm machinery; pumping the water animals need from rivers or deep underground; fuelling live animal transportation in trucks or ships; the constant running of the abattoir's slaughter line; the creation of packaging; and the shipping in refrigerated vehicles of meat products all around the world.

Emissions are further generated through the clearing of land for grazing and to grow animal feed.

There is no polite way to say this, but animals also release a lot of methane through their belches and farts. Methane has a warming effect 86 times more potent than carbon dioxide over a 20-year timeframe.[3] Nitrous oxide emissions – from the breakdown of animal waste – are also released in large quantities, and this compound has almost 300 times the warming impact of carbon dioxide.[4]

With systems of farming varying in different parts of the

world, it is difficult to calculate exactly how much damage animal agriculture causes our planet with its emissions; but in 2006, the United Nations calculated that it was responsible for 18 per cent of the total emissions. In 2009, that figure was revised upwards by two World Bank scientists to 51 per cent. More recently, the Food and Agriculture Organization of the United Nations has stated that animal agriculture is responsible for 14.5 per cent of human-induced emissions.

Despite the variation, all these figures suggest that animal agriculture creates more climate-changing emissions than the entire global transport sector. That's right: animal products are more damaging than every plane, car, truck, train and ship on the planet.[5] It's a sobering thought.

Scientists at Lund University in Sweden came up with four important actions that we should all consider to help reduce climate change; eating a plant-based diet was among them.[6]

WATER

Although the surface of our planet is predominantly water, only three per cent of it is fresh water, and two-thirds of that is held in frozen glaciers or is otherwise unavailable.[7] Already, 1.2 billion people live in areas of water scarcity[8] and, with the world's population predicted to grow to 9.1 billion by 2050, and climate change exacerbating the problem, the strain on this most vital natural, life-preserving resource is only going to increase.[9]

Already, rivers, lakes and aquifers are drying up and more than half of the world's wetlands have disappeared. We would be wise to use water sparingly, and yet global agriculture uses 70 per cent of all available water.[10] And not all agriculture is equal. The thirstiest of all is animal agriculture.

It takes 60 litres of water to produce one pound of potatoes, 229 litres to produce one pound of rice and 9,000 litres to produce one pound of beef.[11] Pigs are said to be the thirstiest animals of all, with the largest farms using water that could supply an entire city.[12]

Rich but water-stressed countries like Saudi Arabia and South Africa recognise the problem and, instead of using their own water resources to grow feed for farmed animals, they rent millions of hectares in Ethiopia, California[13] and elsewhere. It takes the pressure off their own water supplies, but simply exports the problem to other water-stressed regions.[14]

It takes three times more water to produce food for a meat-eater than it does to feed a vegan,[15] and we cannot afford to waste a drop of this precious resource.

POLLUTION

Animal agriculture pollutes our land, waterways and air.

There are billions of farmed animals on this planet, and all of them produce waste. A *lot* of waste. In the days when there was small-scale farming the manure could simply be spread on the land, but we have gone way beyond that recycling of nutrients now. A single dairy cow produces up to 64kg of manure per day[16] and there are one billion cows on the planet.[17] Add to that the billions of other farmed animals – including pigs, sheep, goats, chickens, turkeys, geese, ducks – and it is obvious that the land cannot absorb that much waste. Instead, it is stored in giant, specially built slurry lagoons where, all too often, it leaks out, or overflows and gets into the waterways. Here, it threatens drinking supplies, damages wetlands[18] and fuels 'algal blooms' (rapid accumulation of algae that wipe out aquatic life).[19] Tens of thousands of miles of rivers in the US, Europe and Asia are polluted with slurry each year.[20]

To add to the destruction, noxious gases including ammonia escape these lagoons. Ammonia is a major contributor to acid rain, and two-thirds of man-made ammonia is generated by livestock.[21] It also harms people. Research has shown that those who work inside large-scale factory farms (known in the US as Concentrated Animal Feeding Operations or CAFOs) are more likely to suffer from asthma and respiratory infections.[22] Worldwide, farm workers continue to die from inhalation of methane emitted from the slurry pits.

Not all the waste is stored in lagoons; some is still sprayed onto fields, but there is just too much of it and when large amounts are sprayed, fine dust particles and ammonia are released into the air and carried into the lungs of local residents. In 2015, Dutch researchers found that people living within a kilometre of 15 or more farms had reduced lung function. One of the main culprits they cited was ammonia.[23]

WILDLIFE

Feeding a meat-eating population demands much more land than we'd need to grow food for a vegan population, and this means we must wring every drop of nutrient out of the soil that we possibly can. To this end, 5.6 billion pounds of chemicals are sprayed over the planet each year to kill pests that might harm production.[24] But pests are not all bad. In fact, pests can be very good, and in any case what we call pests the rest of the biological world sees as an inherent part of the ecological system. Without aphids, for example, we don't have larger insects, and without those larger insects we don't have birds.

In the UK, populations of farmland birds have fallen 55 per cent in the past 50 years. The government has stated that these declines are 'largely due to the impact of rapid changes in farmland management', including the intensification of farming, increased pesticide and fertiliser use and the removal of hedgerows.[25]

It's the same across the world. There is an alarming decrease in the number of birds across Europe, with one-third of all species in Germany undergoing a dramatic decline. According to figures released by the German government, species in agricultural areas suffer the worst losses.[26]

Wetland drainage, the conversion of pastureland to crop-land (to grow feed for intensively farmed animals) and overgrazing have meant a loss of 70 per cent of the native

Canadian prairies and a 40 per cent decline in their bird populations since the 1970s.[27]

Australia has one of the highest rates of species extinction in the world [28]. In the state of Queensland alone, 90 per cent of woody vegetation clearing is driven by livestock production[29] and this is estimated to kill more than 30 million native mammals, birds and reptiles every year.[30]

Clearly, it's not just birds under threat. Other wild species are also dying out because of our insatiable desire for meat. A 2016 State of Nature report said: 'The loss of nature in the UK continues . . . The intensification of agriculture has had the biggest impact on wildlife, and this has been overwhelmingly negative.'[31]

Of the 8,688 threatened or near-threatened species worldwide, 63 per cent are threatened by agriculture alone, with the cheetah, the African wild dog and the hairy-nosed otter among the most affected.[32] Agriculture and overexploitation (including fishing) were found to be significantly greater threats to biodiversity than climate change.[33]

DEFORESTATION

Boosting productivity with chemicals will only get us so far. The global demand for meat, milk and eggs means that still more land is needed than is currently available for farming, and we have to get it from somewhere. Inevitably, the farming industry turns its attention to forests and razes them to the ground to make way for grazing or to grow feed for farmed animals. The largest single cause of deforestation is agriculture.[34]

More than half of all tree species in the Amazon – including Brazil nut, wild cacao and acai – are at risk of extinction[35] and the current species losses are just the tip of a terrible iceberg. It takes time for a species to die out after trees are felled, so it is predicted that 80–90 per cent of extinctions caused by damage done between 1970 and 2008 are still to come.[36]

It's not just the Amazon that is being decimated; all forests are under threat. Take the great forests of Sumatra and Borneo, for instance. Once full of tigers, elephants, rhinos and orang-utans, the habitat has been trashed in just one generation.[37] And for what? In large part, it is for palm plantations – a monoculture, doused with herbicides and pesticides that creates a barren landscape and wipes out wild populations.[38] Most of us know that palm products are found in many of the packaged foods on our supermarket shelves; what is less visible is that palm is widely used in animal feed.[39]

Deforestation is devastating for the people and the animals who rely on the habitat. It is also devastating for our planet in its entirety. Trees play a critical role in absorbing greenhouse gas and when they are logged or burned down to clear land for agriculture, huge quantities of climate-changing gases are released into the atmosphere.[40]

Palm oil in plant-based food is a hot topic that is frequently debated on vegan forums. It's your call on how you decide to manage this troublesome ingredient – but you can take comfort in the knowledge that the vegan movement will reduce the need for destructive practices.

The damage caused by deforestation does not end when trees are felled and the animals are driven out of their habitats. Forest soils below the canopy are moist but, without trees to protect them from the sun and the wind, they dry out quickly. The soil becomes more fragile, erodes and can wash away during periods of rain. All too often, the once-rich land becomes barren.

DEPLETED OCEANS

When we think of modern fishing vessels, we may picture the brightly painted recreational boats we see when we visit the coast. Instead, we should conjure up the image of a vessel the length of Buckingham Palace[41 42] or closer to the size of the Sydney Opera House[43] sweeping the oceans and dragging tonnes of sea creatures into nets that are big enough to enclose 13 jumbo jets.[44]

It's little wonder then that more than 85 per cent of the world's fisheries have been pushed beyond their biological limits or are in need of dramatic action to restore them,[45] and whole populations are on the verge of collapse.[46]

This is bad enough, but nets do not discriminate. They drag any species out of the water, whether it is commercially valuable or not. Animals caught unintentionally are known as 'by-catch', and this claims the lives of more than 600,000 marine mammals a year, including whales, dolphins and porpoises;[47] entire species, including the endangered Maui's dolphin and North Atlantic right whale, are being pushed to the brink of extinction. [48, 49]

Sharks,[50] turtles, starfish, sponges and hundreds of thousands of diving seabirds[51] – among them the extraordinary and iconic albatross – are also killed by nets.

It's not just our taste for wild-caught fish that is driving this destruction, it's our taste for farmed fish, as well as meat, milk and eggs. Peruvian anchovies, for example, are taken from the water in their billions[52] but just two per cent of these *anchoveta* are eaten by people, with the remaining 98 per cent reduced to fishmeal or fish oil, which is then added to the feed of farmed animals, including chickens – and fish.[53]

'It is the one decision that has unified the spiritual, physical, mental and emotional side of my humanity. I feel in harmony with animals, and feel that my veganism affirms my desire and commitment to do no harm to animals and the environment. I'm finally living long-held values and morals.'

Jennie R., California, USA

SUSTAINABILITY AND WORLD HUNGER

Until we work out how to colonise Mars, we have just the one planet to live on, and this little orb must sustain billions of people and millions of other species, too. There are finite resources and we need to share them and take care of them. Yet our desire for meat means that not everyone can be fed.

The world already produces enough food to feed every person on the planet and 2.5 billion more[1], yet one in nine people still do not get enough food to be healthy.[2] Meanwhile one-third of the world's cereal harvest and 90 per cent of the world's soya harvest is fed to farmed animals.[3]

It takes more land to produce meat than to produce plant-based foods.[4] This is because animals are inefficient converters of feed to meat. In simple terms, we get back less than we put in. Pigs, for example, require 8.4kg of feed to produce 1kg of meat, while chickens require 3.4kg of feed to produce 1kg.[5] For every 100 calories of grain we feed to farmed animals, we get back only about 40 new calories of milk, 22 calories of eggs, 12 of chicken, 10 of pork or 3 of beef.[6] It's incredibly wasteful and no way to feed a growing population.

The Food and Agriculture Organization of United Nations puts it this way: 'When livestock are raised in intensive systems, they convert carbohydrate and protein that might otherwise be eaten directly by humans and use them to produce a smaller quantity of energy and protein.'[7]

If we were to start from scratch, get our greatest minds round a boardroom table and ask them to devise the best way to use the world's resources and efficiently feed the human population, this plan would be laughed out of the room. No wonder UK think tank Chatham House describes feeding cereals to animals as 'staggeringly inefficient'.[8]

Of course, there are other reasons for hunger – including war, poverty and natural disasters – but there is already enough food for all of us so long as we stop feeding it to farmed animals.

FOR PERSONAL HEALTH

> 'I'd say that within about a week I felt like a different person. I've always had different health problems. I used to have stomach problems. I got a lot of ulcers. I got a lot of acid problems. They cleared up. My mental health was definitely helped. Absolutely give it a go. Why not? It's only a month!'
>
> *Carl Donnelly, comedian, UK*

WHAT VEGANUARY PARTICIPANTS FOUND AFTER 31 DAYS

Each year, people who take part in Veganuary are asked how they found their month of plant-based eating and what physical changes they experienced during that time. Among the most common responses are: my skin cleared up; my digestion is a whole lot better; my sinuses are clearer; my nails are stronger; I have more energy.

Others tell us that they sleep better, have stopped snoring and experience increased libido. For some women, their periods are easier, while one 2017 participant reported an improvement in her menopause symptoms. One person wrote: 'I didn't realise how "sick" my body felt 'til I realised what "healthy" feels like.'

We regularly hear that eczema, psoriasis and acne improve or clear up, and those who suffer irritable bowel syndrome (IBS) often report that the symptoms decrease in severity or disappear altogether. One participant said her chronic fatigue symptoms improved, another that her chronic muscle pain had disappeared. Several people report that their arthritis symptoms eased, with one woman saying, 'My joint pain has gone for the first time in my life.'

Sporty people often find that being vegan helps them recover from training quicker, and that allows them to train even harder and achieve more impressive results. Others are just amazed that they are able to effectively build muscle and endurance on a plant-based diet.

> 'I've never been faster, never been able to recover quicker, never looked better, I've never raced better, I've never been able to go so deep. I went vegan for a challenge, but I stayed vegan because it offered benefits to my life.'
>
> *Dan Geisler, Team GB triathlete*

What is really interesting is the number of people who report better mental clarity, increased concentration and a levelling out of moods. Some participants tell us that their depression symptoms were relieved. For lots of people, eating animal-free foods brings an unexpected contentment, a feeling of inner peace, brought on by eating a diet more in line with their beliefs and principles.

We can't promise everyone that their niggling conditions and chronic illnesses will disappear after 31 days of plant-based eating, but for lots of people, a month without eating animal products brings a stark, often unexpected, improvement.

> ***'Most deaths in the United States are preventable, and they are related to what we eat.'***
>
> Dr Michael Greger, author of *How Not to Die*

HEART DISEASE

Heart disease is the number one cause of death worldwide,[1] and lifestyle factors play a big part. We know, of course, that smoking is bad, that exercise is good and that we should limit alcohol intake and stress. But what about diet?

Research shows that putting plants at the centre of our meals can reduce many of the risk factors for heart disease, including high cholesterol levels, high blood pressure, being overweight and developing type 2 diabetes.

- Elevated blood cholesterol is one risk factor for heart disease. Of meat-eaters, fish-eaters, vegetarians and vegans, vegans have the lowest levels of cholesterol. Animal products contain cholesterol, whereas plant products don't.[2] And it's not just cholesterol in food that causes the problem – it's the amount of saturated fat we eat. Saturated fat causes the liver to produce more cholesterol,[3] and that cholesterol contributes to the formation of plaques, which clog up our arteries, making a heart attack or stroke more likely. High levels of saturated fat are found in processed and fatty meats, hard cheeses, whole milk, cream and butter.[4]

- Another risk factor is high blood pressure, a condition that often cannot be felt, which means there are no warning signs that you may be at risk. Lifestyle factors including diet and exercise are all-important, and once again vegans have been found to have a lower risk.[5]

- A third risk factor is obesity. More than 38 per cent of Americans, 28 per cent of Australians and more than 25 per cent of Britons are obese.[6] It's a serious, life-limiting and life-threatening condition, which makes heart disease and stroke more likely. Studies have regularly shown that vegetarians are slimmer, and vegans appear to have the lowest Body Mass Index of all.[7]

Information on type 2 diabetes – a factor in developing heart disease and a serious condition in its own right – can be found in the next section.

It's never too early to start eating better for your heart, but it seems it is also never too late. Those who have already developed a heart condition may see significant improvements from switching to a plant-based diet.[8]

TYPE 2 DIABETES

Unlike type 1 diabetes, type 2 is largely lifestyle-related, with 80 per cent of those who develop it being overweight.[9]

In his book *How Not to Die*, Dr Michael Greger describes how the condition comes about:

> *'The number of fat cells in your body doesn't change much in adulthood, no matter how much weight you gain or lose. They just swell up with fat as the body gains weight, so when your belly gets bigger, you're not necessarily creating new fat cells; rather you're just cramming more fat into the existing ones. In overweight and obese people, these cells can get so bloated that they actually spill fat back into the bloodstream.'*[10]

Type 2 diabetes is a very serious condition. Complications arising from it include heart disease and stroke, nerve damage, kidney disease, sexual dysfunction, sight loss and blindness, leg ulcers and peripheral vascular disease that can lead to foot or limb amputation. These serious complications are horribly common. In Australia, for example, diabetes is the leading cause of preventable blindness,[11] while in the UK, the number of diabetes-related amputations has reached an all-time high of 20 per day.[12]

Type 2 diabetes is a potentially devastating condition and yet in most people it can be prevented or managed through simple lifestyle changes. In an analysis of 14 available studies, researchers found that 'vegetarians had a 27% lower odds of having diabetes than omnivores' and that 'vegans in particular often had the lowest odds of diabetes when compared to other types of vegetarians'.[13]

The interesting thing is that it isn't just about weight. Even at the same weight as meat-eaters, vegans appear to have less risk of diabetes.[14] This may be down to the difference in fats consumed, but whatever the cause, cutting out animal products and eating plant-based foods reduces the risk of developing this dreadful condition.

And research has shown that with changes to lifestyle, the disease can actually be reversed in 40 per cent of patients.[15]

> 'Plant-based foods, particularly fruit and vegetables, nuts, pulses and seeds, have been shown to help in the treatment of many chronic diseases and are often associated with lower rates of Type 2 diabetes, less hypertension, lower cholesterol levels and reduced cancer rates.'[16]
>
> *Diabetes UK*

CANCERS

In 2015, World Health Organisation scientists felt they had amassed enough evidence from decades of work to state categorically that processed red meat causes cancer, while red meat is a 'probable' cause.[17] This means that bacon, sausages, hot dogs, ham, salami and pepperoni are now officially classified as carcinogens, just as tobacco is.[18] They warned that eating 50g of processed red meat a day – that's less than two slices of bacon – raises the risk of colon cancer by 18 per cent.[19] Immediately after the announcement, sales of bacon and sausages fell sharply.[20]

It's not just the meat itself but how it's cooked that can cause trouble. Whenever meat – including beef, chicken and fish – is cooked at high temperatures, chemicals called heterocyclic amines (HCAs) form, and these are also carcinogenic.[21] The longer meat is cooked, the more HCAs form, and this may explain why eating well-done meat is associated with increased risk of breast, colon, oesophagus, lung, pancreatic, prostate and stomach cancer.[22] Of course, *not* cooking meat thoroughly is connected to a greater risk of food-borne infections and food poisoning[23] so there is risk in meat-eating either way.

'Recent scientific studies have suggested that dairy products may be linked to an increased risk for prostate cancer and testicular cancer.'[24] This may be down to dairy consumption boosting the hormone IGF-1 (insulin-like growth factor 1) in the bloodstream, but there are other possible mechanisms being studied and more work is needed to show a conclusive link.

> It's the position of the Academy of Nutrition and Dietetics that appropriately planned vegetarian, including vegan, diets are healthful, nutritionally adequate and may provide health benefits for the prevention and treatment of certain diseases. Vegetarians and vegans are at reduced risk of certain health conditions, including ischemic heart disease, type 2 diabetes, hypertension, certain types of cancer, and obesity.[25]
>
> *The Academy of Nutrition and Dietetics*

FOR GLOBAL HEALTH

DISEASES FROM FARMED ANIMALS

Damaging as animal products can be to our own health, this is nothing compared with what the industry could do to human health at a global level. Did you know that many of the common diseases that make us sick originated in animals we farmed? It is thought that smallpox came from camelpox, measles from the rinderpest virus in cows, whooping cough from pigs, leprosy from water buffalo, the common cold from horses and influenza from poultry.[1] It seems animal farming has been harming us for centuries!

One hundred years ago, half the world's population was infected with a particularly nasty flu virus, which killed up to 100 million people. Sad to say, this isn't old news and the threat remains. Flu viruses are still around, always mutating, always looking for ways to get stronger and to spread further, and factory farms with high densities of animals with already compromised immune systems[2] provide the ideal environment for new strains to evolve.[3]

If we want to stop new diseases and new strains of existing diseases emerging, we would do well to move away from farming animals.

ANTIBIOTICS

Intensive farming is a practice that stresses animals and weakens their immune systems while simultaneously exposing them to squalor. No surprise, then, that disease on such farms is rife. But instead of providing better conditions, the industry doses the animals with antibiotics.

Antibiotics are the wonder drugs that changed modern medicine and have saved countless human lives since their discovery less than one hundred years ago. But we've become complacent. We take them when we don't need them, or don't finish the prescribed course. And we add them to the feed of farmed animals, whether they need them or not, often just because of their growth-promoting qualities. By over-using them like this, we have allowed resistant strains of superbugs to emerge.

Dame Sally Davies, the Chief Medical Officer for England, has warned of an 'apocalyptic scenario' where diseases become resistant to all our types of antibiotics. Dr Margaret Chan, former Director-General of the World Health Organisation, has said 'we face a post-antibiotic era, in which many common infections will no longer have a cure and, once again, kill unabated'. The British government talks about 'ten million deaths per year' if something is not done.[4]

In the US, it is estimated that around 70 per cent of all antibiotics used are fed to pigs, poultry and cows.[5] In Australia, data is less easy to come by and industry secrecy about antibiotic use has been blamed for undermining efforts to prevent superbugs developing.[6] In the European Union, use of antibiotics for non-medicinal purposes, including adding them to animal feed, has been banned since 2006,[7] and the amount of antibiotics given to farmed animals in the UK has slowly been dropping in recent years. But animals are still given the drugs in substantial quantities, and this threatens all of our futures. The situation is so serious that in 2016 the United Nations General Assembly held a meeting involving all 193 member states to discuss solutions.[8]

What can individuals do? We can use antibiotics only when we really need them and ensure we finish the course, and we can stop eating animal products. Even organic meat, milk and eggs can come from animals who have been given antibiotics.[9]

FOR THE ADVENTURE

There are lots of great reasons to try vegan for 31 days. Most people will say they are doing it for the animals, for the environment or for their own health. But some people do it just because. For them it is a challenge, to see what it would be like, to see if they can do it and to see how their life might change.

For everyone, though, there is a period of adjustment – of learning, finding new foods and recipes and sometimes discovering new ways of cooking. Almost everyone reports that, where they had expected to feel more limited in their food choices, instead a whole new world of amazing ingredients opens up before them.

Research shows that most of us cook just nine different meals on a repetitive loop, even though we may own several recipe-packed cookbooks.[1] We get stuck in a rut, and as a result we lose all passion for our food. It's easily done. After all – which of us, when walking through the supermarket aisle, stops to pick up dudhi, samphire or okra to use in a midweek meal?

Vegans. That's who!

> 'There is so much variety out there, and I think my taste buds have changed since I eat so much more fresh wholefoods – food just tastes that much better.'
>
> *Emily J., London, UK, Veganuary Class of 2017*

OK, so not all vegans create exotic dishes and even those who do probably don't do so every day of the week, but people who take part in Veganuary often say that the culinary shake-up means they are trying foods they have never tried before. They are making new meals and rediscovering their love of great food. But they also find that shops are full of vegan convenience foods, so on the days when they feel like pie and mashed potato, that's exactly what they can have.

The fact that 99 per cent of people who take part in Veganuary would recommend it to others shows just how much fun those 31 days can be. The most common response to the question: *What advice would you give to someone thinking about trying vegan for 31 days*? is: *Do it. There is nothing to lose and so much to gain.*

'My advice for people thinking about trying veganism is: go do it! If January is when you've got that extra power, and you can join the Veganuary community and get it done, then try it and it will be the best decision you ever made.'

Tim Shieff, professional free runner, UK

SO, WHAT WILL I ACHIEVE?

'It's like having an epiphany and to begin with you want to shout what you have learned from the roof-tops. I have made some great friends online, I have made some great friends in the 'free-from' aisle in my local supermarket! I'm 28 pounds lighter and now run three times a week as part of my vegan running club. To say it has improved several aspects of my life for the better would be an understatement!'

Laura-Jayne W., Shropshire, UK,
Veganuary Class of 2017

Everyone who tries vegan for 31 days gets something different out of it. For some, their health improves radically. The niggles, illnesses and conditions they once experienced clear up, and they are left with a new vigour, a newfound confidence and a much brighter future. Amateur and professional athletes report training benefits and say they wish they had done it sooner.

Lots of people lose weight, which is great if they needed to. Those whose weight is on the low side, too, are often pleased to see they can make these dietary changes without losing additional weight.

But not everyone will notice an instantaneous, miraculous change. For some people, the fact that *nothing* changes is what is so great – they can still cook tasty food, feel the same as they did before and can still eat out with friends in local restaurants. They're just doing it all plant-based.

Those who have struggled with the realities of animal farming – perhaps they have seen reports in newspapers or online about the treatment of animals – say they feel that a weight has been lifted from them. They never wanted to be part of the cruelty, but they did not know how to separate themselves from it. For them, a clearer conscience changes their whole outlook on life. Bringing practice in line with principles is also a wonderful outcome for those concerned about our planet, its wild spaces and its inhabitants.

One interesting consequence is that some people say they feel more connection with nature. Understanding the impact of our food choices inevitably rings some alarm bells, but it also makes us more aware of how beautiful and fragile this planet is. Lots of people say they enjoy being out in nature more, and they feel a greater sense of connection, empathy and even compassion, which spills into every part of their lives.

There are so many possible outcomes and we can't say for sure how being vegan will change *your* life. There is only one way to find that out.

HOW TO GO VEGAN

• • •

This is the big question – how exactly do we make this change in our lives? Since most of us were brought up eating meat, milk and eggs, it's natural to wonder about what we'll miss when leaving these products behind. But going vegan doesn't have to feel like a huge sacrifice. In fact, it really should not feel anything like that at all!

Some people – but not all – find that it's easier to switch one product at a time, so it doesn't seem like an overwhelming overhaul of their diet. They may try various brands of meat-free sausages or burgers to start with, then decide to stick to one that they like best. They may find that the faux fish fingers taste just like real fish, and start to include these in their diet before switching to dairy-free yoghurts and milks. Whether you're a toe-dipper or a cannonballer into the world of veganism, you can get the taste you love without the animal suffering, cholesterol and poor environmental record. You just need to know where to look!

Like all new habits and lifestyles, there will be a period of adjustment while you learn which foods are vegan and where to find them, but it really won't take long before you're veganing like a pro. There is not space in this book to share with you all the great vegan brands and products you can find in your local shops, but what we can do is give you some good general tips. Then it's over to you to do a little research of your own.

Before we get started, a brief word of advice about putting pressure on yourself: please don't. If you're keen to try veganism but find you fall off the wagon, don't assume that veganism is not for you. You just made a mistake. That's OK, we're all human. Just start again. Every day you eat plant-based is a wonderful thing, so don't worry too much about the odd hiccup.

WHAT TO DO FIRST

The last thing you want to do is wake up on 1 January – or whatever date you've chosen to start your vegan odyssey – and find there's nothing for breakfast but dry bread and black tea. With such a desperate start to the day, you'll come to the rapid conclusion that veganism sucks, and we'd be surprised if you were still vegan at lunchtime. With just a little planning, though, you'll find that a vegan breakfast can be surprisingly similar to a non-vegan one. So before you begin, ask yourself this: *What do I normally eat for breakfast?*

If cereal is your thing, you'll find that lots of cereals are vegan, but you will need to watch out for honey and switch to a plant-based milk. There are so many non-dairy milks available now – including soya, oat, rice, hemp, coconut, almond and cashew – and different tastes suit different people. It's true that none of them taste exactly like cows' milk because they're not the same thing, and we only drink cows' milk in any case because that's what we're used to. You'll need a little time to get used to a new milk, too. Experiment a bit until you find the ones you like best. It may be that almond is perfect for your coffee but you prefer oat on your cereal. Mix it up, and see what works for you.

If you like toast, you'll find most breads are vegan and dairy-free spreads are available in virtually every mainstream shop as well as in many health food shops. Jam, marmalade, peanut butter and yeast extracts like Marmite are all vegan anyway, so your toast need never be naked.

You'll find dairy-free yoghurts are readily available, and most people can't tell them apart from the dairy versions. Top them off with nuts, seeds and fruit. Fruit is good – eat lots! And why not allow your newly found adventurous spirit to lead you to the fruits you've never picked up in the supermarket before? You know the ones – those weirdly shaped, hairy, spiky, slightly scary ones? Some are an acquired taste but most taste beautiful.

If you're a Big Breakfast Person, that's good, too. Hash browns and baked beans are fine. Add in some vegan sausages and vegan bacon, and top up with tomatoes and mushrooms or avocado. You can even make scrambled tofu if you'd like, and it is surprisingly similar to scrambled egg.

And don't worry – ketchup is vegan, too, as are coffee, tea and fruit juices.

So, you've had a three-course breakfast and your day is off to a flying start. But unless you want to eat the same foods for *every* breakfast, lunch and dinner, you'll need to branch out. Our advice in those first few days is not to get too radical. If you normally eat soup for lunch, find a vegan soup to enjoy. If you like a casserole for your dinner, make a vegan version. There will be plenty of time to don an apron and create avocado gazpacho with Egyptian dukkah dust but for now, there's nothing wrong with sticking to what you know.

If you're not sure whether a product you normally buy is vegan, check out the label-reading section in this book. You can also search online, or ask within the Veganuary Facebook group, and if you're still not sure, contact Veganuary and we'll do our best to find out. Whatever you do, please don't give up just because you don't know whether your favourite sandwich pickle is vegan. (By the way, it probably is.)

VEGAN AT HOME

SURPRISINGLY VEGAN FOODS

The biggest concern for people contemplating a vegan diet is almost always: *What will I eat?* There is a notion that there are specialist vegan products that taste like cardboard and are only found on dusty shelves in out-of-the-way shops, and that all the old favourites must be relinquished. This is very far from the truth.

Take a look inside any meat-eater's kitchen and you'll find a great number of everyday store-cupboard products that are already vegan. They weren't designed for vegans, but they contain no animal products at all, and include items we eat regularly and couldn't imagine life without. Peanut butter, yeast extracts, jams and marmalades, baked beans, dried pasta, rice, almost all bread, many types of gravy granules, vegetable stock cubes, chopped tomatoes, oven chips and hash browns, coconut milk, lots of curry pastes, many breakfast cereals, herbs, spices, tomato ketchup and HP sauce, mustard and pickles, olive oil and vegetable oils, soy sauce, fruit juice, tea and coffee, lots of cookies, crackers, crispbreads and crisps, and of course fruit and vegetables – fresh, dried, tinned and frozen. All vegan.

That's a pretty good start, isn't it?

Having so many everyday products already free from animal parts means that we can make small, almost unnoticeable changes to our existing diet that will transform it from an omnivorous one to a vegan one. We can ease ourselves into veganism with beans on toast (we need only change the margarine) or sausages and mash (just choose veggie sausages and vegetable gravy), and it won't seem like the world has shifted beneath our feet. The meal is essentially the same; it's just a different brand of the same product.

And there are a lot of vegan products out there – from croissants and cookies to pretzels and pies. Check out veganuary.com and look elsewhere online for 'accidentally vegan products' and you'll see just how many there are. If you're craving something and don't know where to look, ask the Veganuary Facebook group – if anyone knows, you'll find the answer there! Think of it as the oracle for all things vegan.

Being vegan doesn't have to mean a whole new way of life. In most cases, it is simply a question of knowing which brands are vegan and choosing those. Quite often, the brand you've been buying all along was vegan anyway. You just didn't know it.

Do bear in mind that you may need to alter your shopping habits slightly and you'll soon learn that it's better to be prepared. In many areas, you're unlikely to track down vegan cheese at the neighbourhood convenience store and you may need to travel to a supermarket further afield, rely on a health-food store with limited opening hours or search for key ingredients online. You might sacrifice some convenience, but gain some awesome organisational skills!

READING LABELS

We won't lie to you. In the first fortnight of being vegan, you are going to read a LOT of food labels and your weekly shop is likely to take just that little bit longer. When you start to look at ingredients, you may be shocked to find you have no idea what half of them are, or why you are eating them. *I mean, what is 'casein' and what's it doing in my cracker, and what do you mean I've been eating crushed beetles?*

Since it's better to know what we're putting into our bodies than to go on in ignorance, reading labels at this stage is a good thing, and it won't be for ever. Very soon you'll be fluent in this new language, and will just pick up one brand over another without having to check each time. You'll know that D2 is vegan but D3 may not be. You'll know that whey is from milk, and aspic can be made from clarified meat. You'll even know what isinglass is. Just imagine how many people you will wow at dinner parties.

Here are a few tips to get you started when you pick up a package off the shelf.

1. Does it say 'Vegan' on the packaging? Yes? Read no further.

2. Does it say 'Vegetarian' on the package? Yes? That's a good start, but let's examine it more closely. In the UK, across Europe and in the US, Canada and Australia, ingredients that are likely to cause allergies must be declared on the package. These major allergens include milk, egg and fish ingredients. This means if it says it's vegetarian and these allergens are *not* listed, then (providing it doesn't contain any E numbers, which may require further inspection – see below) there is just one more check to make. Is there honey in it? No? Great! It's vegan.

3. Not all companies label things as well as they might. In this case, you will need your forensic head on, and to look at those ingredients separately. At this point, it is common to wonder how such a small package can contain so many ingredients. It can be quite a revelation that the natural, healthy diet we thought we had contains all manner of items we can't identify. Here are some hidden demons to look out for:

    - **Albumen/albumin** – from eggs, and may be used in baked goods

    - **Aspic** – an industry alternative to gelatine, and usually made from meat or fish

- **Carmine/cochineal/E120** – the red pigment of crushed female cochineal beetles, used as a food colouring in cakes and sweets

- **Casein** – a protein from milk, may be found in soups, chocolate and baked goods

- **E numbers** – in Europe, E numbers are a feature of many ingredient lists and some of them are animal derived. You can find a list of non-vegan E numbers on veganuary.com, so you know what to look out for

- **Gelatine** – obtained by boiling the skin, tendons, ligaments and bones of cows or pigs, and found in jelly, chewy sweets, cakes and in the capsules of some vitamins

- **Honey** – food for bees, made by bees. Often found in breakfast cereals and cereal bars

- **Isinglass** – derived from the swim bladders of fish, and used in the clarification of some wines and beers. (You won't find this ingredient on a label, though, as strictly speaking it is not an ingredient but a product used in the process. Visit www.barnivore.com for a list of vegan wine, beer and spirits)

- **Lactose** – a sugar from milk, can be found in baked goods

- **Lard** – white pork fat that has been rendered and clarified

- **Propolis** – used by bees in the construction of their hives. May be found in foods claiming specific health benefits

- **Shellac** – the resin secreted by female lac insects, and used as a food glaze

- **Vitamin D3** – it's possible to get vegan Vitamin D3, but often it comes from the liver of fish. If the pack says 'vegetarian', you'll know which one you have

- **Whey** – the liquid remaining after milk has been curdled and strained. Often found in baked products

4. If you're not a fan of reading labels (believe us, some people are!) or are short on time, you can use an app such as Spoon Guru to check products – set your dietary requirement and get scanning to find out what is safe. Not every product is in the database (that would be a tall order), but more are being added every day.

5. If you're really not sure, go online. There are thousands of vegans on social media – including in the Veganuary Facebook group – who will know the answer immediately. Not only will they be able to tell you whether your product is vegan, they will be able to suggest a heap of similar products, too. So, when we say becoming vegan opens up whole new areas of food rather than restricting options, we're not kidding.

6. If all else fails, contact the manufacturer. If your favourite brand isn't vegan, contact them anyway and ask why not. Ingredients change all the time, and if a company realises it will sell more by substituting an animal ingredient for a vegan version, it will listen. It may take some time, but it will definitely listen.

Here are three more tips to help you on your way.

1. Don't believe that 'dairy-free' or 'lactose-free' means vegan. Sometimes it does; sometimes it doesn't. It's best to check to see what other ingredients are in there.

2. Lactic acid is vegan. Lactose is not. It's a bit confusing but it's great news for fans of pickles.

3. This may seem confusing, but if a package says 'may contain traces of milk and eggs', it could still be vegan. In some countries, it's mandatory to give this warning if the

product has been made in a factory where non-vegan items have been handled. In other countries, it's a voluntary statement. Either way, it doesn't affect whether the product is vegan. It may help to think of it like this – imagine a friend is making you a vegan sandwich in their kitchen. Just because they've previously prepared non-vegan food in that kitchen, doesn't make the sandwich any less vegan. Be sure to check the ingredient and the allergen lists to see what is actually *in* the product – unless you have an allergy or intolerance, you can disregard these 'cross-contamination' warnings.

VEGAN INGREDIENT ESSENTIALS

While having a kitchen full of versatile and tasty ingredients will be your first step towards making fantastic vegan food, don't feel that you need to rush out in search of white truffle oil this instant. You already have many of the basics in your kitchen, so use this section as a guide to help grow your vegan larder over time.

PROTEIN SOURCES

- **Tofu:** Choose firmer varieties for cooking or silken for sauces and desserts. Plain tofu will soak up flavours and there are many varieties that are already flavoured or marinated

- **Seitan:** A high-protein meat replacement made from wheat gluten, which has a great 'meaty' texture

- **Tempeh:** Similar to tofu in that it's made from fermented soya beans, but firmer and with a stronger flavour. Try marinating it

- **Peas:** Garden peas or petit pois, frozen or tinned

- **Beans:** Choose from a wide variety, including kidney, cannellini, pinto, black, lima and chickpeas (garbanzo). There are ready-to-eat tinned beans and dried versions that you will need to soak before cooking

- **Lentils:** Puy, red, brown or green. Buy them dried or in pre-packed form, and use them in sauces, stews, curries, bolognese, shepherd's pie, lasagne and whatever else you like

- **Seeds:** Sunflower, pumpkin, sesame, chia, flax. Seeds are packed full of good stuff! Great on cereals, in stir-frys, salads, stews – in fact pretty much anywhere

- **Nuts:** Almonds, cashews, walnuts, Brazils, pine nuts, pistachios, peanuts

- **Nut butters:** You probably already have peanut butter,

but did you know you can get others? Almond, cashew and hazelnut are all really tasty

DAIRY REPLACEMENTS

- **Vegetable spread:** Look for the range of dairy-free butters in supermarkets and health food shops. Be aware of buttermilk in the ingredients – that's not vegan

- **Dairy-free cheese:** There are many brands and flavours available to try, including hard cheeses, grated and cream cheeses. Tastes vary – if you don't like the first ones you try, keep trying others!

- **Plant milks:** Try soya, almond, rice, hemp, almond, coconut, cashew and various flavoured milks. We love unsweetened almond milk on cereals

- **Yoghurts:** Some are made from soya, others from coconut, and they come in a wide range of flavours

- **Ice cream:** There are ever-growing ranges of vegan ice creams, cones and choc ices in many different flavours. And the big ice cream brands you already know and love are getting in on the act too!

- **Cream:** There are vegan single creams for pouring on desserts or using in soups, whipping cream for cakes and squirty cream in a can for anything you like!

GRAINS

- **Rice:** Choose from brown, white, basmati, jasmine or wild

- **Quinoa:** A high-protein grain that can be used like rice

- **Couscous:** Made from wheat, and available in white, wholewheat and flavoured varieties. Ready in minutes and delicious hot or cold

- **Pasta:** Avoid egg pasta and any coloured with squid ink. Otherwise, all shapes and sizes are good

- **Polenta:** Cornmeal that can be made into porridge/ oatmeal, turned into a traditional Mediterranean bake or eaten as a great alternative to mashed potato

- **Oats and millet:** Excellent choices for a hearty breakfast

BAKING

- **Egg replacer:** There are several brands available online and in health food shops; just follow the instructions

- **Flax seeds:** Can be used as an egg replacer. One tablespoon of ground flax seeds with three tablespoons of warm water replaces one egg

- **Chia seeds:** Another egg replacer. One tablespoon of seeds with two tablespoons of water replaces one egg

- **Coconut oil:** Good for replacing butter

- **Agave nectar:** Great instead of honey

- **Maple syrup:** Another honey replacement

- **Blackstrap molasses:** A great binding agent for homemade flapjacks, granola and power bars. A fantastic source of iron

- **Pastry:** Some of the leading ready-made puff and shortcrust pastry brands are vegan if you don't fancy making your own

CONDIMENTS AND SAUCES

- **Miso:** A traditional Japanese seasoning. Eat as a soup or use as a flavouring

- **Tamari and soy sauce:** Tamari is a thicker, less salty, fermented sauce that contains less wheat than soy sauce

- **Table sauces:** Including barbecue, Thai sweet chilli, ketchup, HP, mint and apple sauces, chutneys and mustards

HEALTHY SNACKS

- **Dried fruit:** Choose from pineapple, mangos, strawberries and a host of other fruits. Eat them fresh, too

- **Hummus:** The vegan's friend! A range of flavours and styles available. Perfect for picnics, sandwiches and dipping vegetable sticks into

- **Fruit and cereal bars:** Raw fruit bars and baked cereal bars. Just look out for honey

- **Popcorn:** Lots of flavours and brands are vegan – or it's fun to make your own

- **Nuts and seeds:** Always a handy snack to keep in your bag

- **Dark chocolate:** There is iron to be found in dark chocolate, so never feel guilty!

VEGETABLES

Don't hold back here, eat a rainbow every day.

EASY REPLACEMENTS

The simplest way to begin your vegan adventure is to stick to your favourite, tried-and-tested recipes and veganise them by making simple substitutions.

On cereal and in coffee, try different plant milks until you find the ones that suit you best. On toast, pick a dairy-free spread; you will barely notice the difference. And there are many instances where you can swap cheese, ice cream and cream for the dairy-free versions and no one would be any the wiser.

Here's how to veganise a week of popular evening meals.

1. Spaghetti bolognese

Use your favourite recipe, and just use soya mince/soy grounds or lentils instead of the meat. If you'd normally use meat stock, replace with vegetable stock. Use dairy-free margarine or olive oil on the pasta instead of butter. Vegan Parmesan can be found in some supermarkets, in health food shops and online.

2. Burgers

There are loads of vegan burgers/patties available; just use an egg-free mayonnaise. Ketchup, mustard and pickles are usually already vegan, and you'll find that most bread buns are vegan too (except pesky brioche buns, which contain egg). Fancy a cheeseburger? Just use a vegan cheese slice or two – pick one that melts well.

3. **Chilli con carne** (you'd better now call it chilli *non* carne!) Another simple substitution! Just use soya mince/soy grounds instead of the meat, or use brown lentils if you prefer. If you're using stock, use a vegetable one. Often the pre-mixed chilli spices are vegan. We like to put red wine and a dash of cocoa powder in ours!

4. **Lasagne**
For the meat layer, follow the same pattern as for the bolognese sauce or the chilli, and use soya mince/soy grounds or lentils. For the white sauce, use dairy-free milk and spread. Classicists won't add cheese to a lasagne sauce but if you like it, go ahead and add grated vegan cheese or nutritional yeast flakes. Dried lasagne sheets generally don't contain egg – but fresh ones often do.

5. **Fajitas**
Replace the meat strips with vegan meat strips! Some of the fajita kits are already vegan, so you need do nothing else except whip up a guacamole; and either leave out the sour cream and cheese or use vegan versions of each.

6. **Mac and cheese**
Swap the milk for plant milk and the cheese for a melting

vegan cheese – you could add nutritional yeast if you like it extra cheesy. That's it!

7. **Pizza**
   If you make the dough yourself, the chances are you're already making a vegan pizza base. If you buy the dough or base, just check that no milk proteins have been added. Add your favourite toppings, including faux ham or salami, and cover with a dairy-free cheese. Make sure the one you buy melts properly.

> 'I've learned so many new things and cooking techniques that I would never have tried before. Anything you love as a non-vegan you can make vegan.'
>
> *Christelle R., Alberta, Canada,*
> *Veganuary Class of 2016*

THE ONLY VEGAN IN THE FAMILY

If you're the only one in your household trying vegan at this time, that doesn't have to be a problem, but if you're young and living at home, you may have to clear another hurdle before your vegan adventure can begin. We know that not everyone's families are as supportive as the fledgling vegan might hope, but this is not because they just like making life hard. It's often because they don't know much about veganism, and they worry about their loved one's health or having to make two separate meals after a long day at work, or how these changes will impact the weekly shopping bill.

If you want to try veganism but are faced with opposition at home, we'd suggest you talk it through as calmly as possible to find out what the reasons are. The sections in this book should help you counter any concerns about health, nutrition and cost, but if the problem lies with having to cook additional meals every day, then it's clear some practicalities will need to be ironed out.

First, if you don't normally help with shopping and cooking this would be a very good time to start! It might be stretching the family bonds just a little too far to expect someone else to do your research, read labels, discover new products and recipes and then cook them for you. Time to step up!

You may find there needs to be a little bargaining at this stage: *I'll cook a vegan meal for everyone twice a week if you make sure the other meals can be veganised, too.*

This doesn't have to be as complex as it might sound! It might be as simple as adding different toppings to a pizza base, or cooking up plant-based sausages, burgers or a pie alongside the meaty ones. So long as the accompaniments are vegan, or can be removed before someone adds butter or cheese, then this approach shouldn't feel like an extra burden. For something like a stir-fry, simply use the same ingredients split between two pans, then add meat to one and tofu or vegan meaty strips into the other.

Obviously, it will take a little adjusting for everyone, but that's why we suggest people try it for 31 days. That's a great introduction time for everyone to get used to it, and for it to become something like second nature, but if there is still resistance, you might like to throw in some washing-up duties. Some might call that bribery, but if it works . . .

If you're the main cook in your house, or a regular cook, things are usually a lot easier, and the rest of your family will almost certainly be happy with at least some of your veganised versions of your family favourites. With meals like chilli and bolognese, there's a good chance that no one will be able to tell the difference anyway. If the others want to add dairy cheese on top when you add vegan cheese, that's not going to cause any problems.

Even so, there may be times when someone in your household just wants meat or cheese, and there will be no talking them out of it. We can't force others to be vegan, after all. Perhaps you can agree on a set number of vegan meals for everyone each week and then compromise on the others, although whether you will want to cook meat when you're trying out veganism is up to you.

Often when people are drawn into plant-based eating by a member of their household trying vegan they find that the new way of eating suits them better than they expected. They are surprised that there are meaty chunks that can be used in casseroles, stews and curries, for example, and 'meat' slices that are great instead of chicken and ham in sandwiches. There are 'chicken' pies, 'beef' pasties, fishless fingers and even vegan haggis – an ever-growing range of great-tasting products that everyone can enjoy.

How you manage the meals if you are the only vegan in the family will depend on who normally cooks, the type of foods you make and how far the rest of your household is willing to go along with your food choices. Usually, some compromise is required, and some sharing of the cooking to ensure everybody is happy. In many cases, if the household's main cook goes vegan, the whole family tends to eat vegan at home. Chef's rules!

DOES BEING VEGAN COST MORE?

Being vegan absolutely doesn't have to create additional expense and, in fact, depending on the kinds of products you buy and how much cooking you do, it can be a lot cheaper than buying animal products. Most store-cupboard essentials – like pasta, rice, potatoes, beans, tinned tomatoes, lentils and fresh seasonal or frozen veggies – are cheap, and you're likely to be buying those already anyway.

Besides, meat is *really* expensive. A joint of meat or a piece of fish is probably the most pricey thing you will buy in a supermarket outside of the alcohol aisle. And the price you pay for meat and other animal products is not even the full cost, which is huge when we consider the health and environmental implications, plus the subsidies that taxpayers contribute to the farming and slaughter of animals.

But what you want to know is: will going vegan blow the weekly budget? And the answer is: most people find little overall difference. Some products, like dairy-free cheeses and milks, are more expensive than the dairy versions, but then there are some premium dairy brands that are more expensive still. It depends on what you used to buy.

If we compare like for like, we can see, for example, that the price of vegan sausage rolls in one UK supermarket falls right in the middle of the range of the prices for meat-based sausage rolls. And the fishless fingers, while coming towards the top end of the range in terms of cost, are not as expensive as some of the premium fish brands.

If you have traditionally bought foodstuffs at the lower end of the pricing scale, choosing vegan products might be a greater expense than you are used to, but the overall basket price is still likely to stay the same or come down. This is because of the greater amount of fruit and veg you'll be buying and enjoying as a vegan, and the fact that you won't be buying meat. And those who used to buy joints of meat, whole organic chickens or premium dairy brands will almost certainly see the cost of their shopping basket decrease.

No matter what you eat, there are ways to help keep the budget down, including cooking from scratch rather than buying processed or pre-packaged foods, bulk-buying staples such as rice and pasta and cooking up batches of food to freeze for future use.

If you're on a budget, visit the Recipes section of the Veganuary website, where there is a part dedicated to cheap vegan meal ideas. You could also check out Jack Monroe's *Cooking on a Bootstrap* blog, where you'll find lots more delicious cheap vegan recipes.

And if you're eating out, you'll see that the vegan options on menus are almost always cheaper than the meat-based meals.

VEGAN OUT IN THE WORLD

EATING OUT

Once upon a time, a vegan wandering alone and hungry on the high street would have no choice but to buy an apple or a bag of ready salted potato crisps to satisfy the pangs, and wait until they got home before they could eat properly. These days, it's possible to get a choice of vegan meals almost anywhere, with restaurant chains vying with one another to offer the widest range and the most exciting dishes. From burgers and burritos to sandwiches and sushi, vegan food is plentiful, varied and just round the corner.

CHAIN RESTAURANTS

In the UK, vegans will find great options at Zizzi, Pizza Express, Wagamama, All Bar One, Wetherspoon, Las Iguanas, Carluccio's, Yo! Sushi, Pret a Manger, Ask, Leon, the

Handmade Burger Company and even Nando's, McDonald's and Toby Carvery.

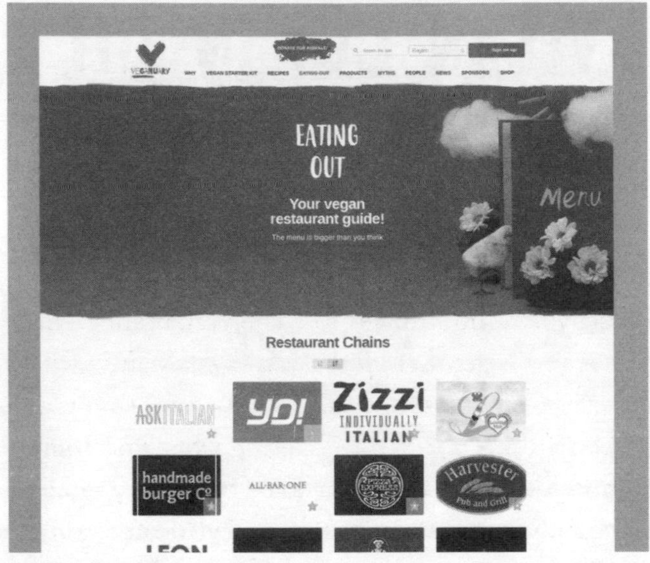

The eating out section on the Veganuary website has all the most up-to-date information about vegan options at independent and chain restaurants.

In the US, look out for options at The Daily Grill, Del Taco, The Cheesecake Factory, Chipotle, Denny's, Jason's Deli, Kona Grill, Little Caesars Pizza, Papa John's, Starbucks, Taco Bell, Veggie Grill and Native Foods.

In Canada, try Teriyaki Experience, Hero Burger, Harvey's, Extreme Pita, Just Falafel, Subway, Magic Oven, Panago Pizza, Chipotle, Taco Bell and Tim Hortons.

While in Australia, head to Montezuma's, Sushi Train, Sumo Salad, Subway, Indian Brothers, Domino and Lord of the Fries.

One other international restaurant chain to look out for is Loving Hut – it's 100 per cent vegan, and its restaurants can be found in 35 countries, from England to Australia, from Taiwan to the USA.

VEGGIE AND VEGAN RESTAURANTS

Of course, you're not limited to chain restaurants. There are now so many vegetarian and vegan restaurants, with new ones opening every week, that a host of new eating options will suddenly open up for you. Wherever you are in the world, your best options will be in the cities, but there are plenty of meat-free restaurants opening in smaller towns, too.

From fast food cafes to raw food restaurants to gourmet plant-based dining, you'll find your best local options at Vanilla-Bean.com or HappyCow.net. These websites, and their apps, list thousands of restaurants, cafes and health food stores all over the world, and are updated regularly. And they don't just list specifically vegan restaurants – they list all the restaurants they know of where a vegan meal can be found.

INDEPENDENT RESTAURANTS

With more and more independent restaurants catering for vegans, there is every chance that your favourite eatery will already have – or will happily create – plant-based meals for you.

If you know you're going to a restaurant where you haven't been before – or haven't been since you went vegan – it's wise to call ahead and speak to the chef so you're not left hungry when you visit. It's rare to find a chef who won't prepare a meal for you, and often they relish the challenge of cooking something different from their usual offerings. If you are going to a large get-together, such as a family gathering or a work dinner, it's worth letting the organiser know that you'll speak to the venue directly beforehand. That way you can be sure that messages won't get lost or confused, and vital facts won't go missing along the way.

Even if you're not able to call ahead, don't worry; you can still make requests once you're inside the restaurant. By being vegan, you're not being a bore or a burden. You're a customer, and customers make requests *all the time*, for all sorts of reasons, so go ahead and ask for a dish to be altered to suit you. You may be amazed at what a chef can whip up – but if they struggle, then putting a few side dishes together can work surprisingly well!

If you're out with a group and feel a little self-conscious about querying menu items at the table, simply excuse yourself before ordering and have a quiet word with your server. This is also a great way to ask about ingredients, as the waiting staff may need to check with the kitchen, and this can delay the ordering process. You might want to know whether they cook with butter or vegetable oil, if the pasta they use is made with egg, or if the garlic mushrooms can be prepared without cream. And you might find it much easier to ask a few questions when you haven't got (what feels like) a hundred pairs of eyes on you.

A word of warning: although veganism is much more widely understood than ever before, don't assume that all restaurant staff know what it is. Politely explain what you do and don't eat, and take the time to answer their questions. You might say something like, 'I'm vegan, so I don't eat eggs, milk or cheese. I was wondering whether you know if your pizza dough has any milk or eggs in it, and if I can get the Vegetariana without cheese?' You may be the first vegan they've met – so a little patience and politeness will go a long way, and it may just score you a bigger portion. Increasingly, though, serving staff and chefs know exactly what to offer, because they get asked all the time. Besides, all good chefs will know which allergens are in their food – and this handily includes eggs, milk products and shellfish.

Whether your restaurant has done itself proud or could use a little encouragement, Veganuary can help support and create more vegan options in your area. We produce business cards that you can leave on the table after your meal. One states: **Thank you for your vegan options!** The other: **I wish you had more vegan options**, with the text directing the restaurant to a free catering guide and recipe pack.

I wish you had
MORE VEGAN OPTIONS!
For a free catering guide and additional support to improve your vegan options, please contact
restaurants@veganuary.com
VEGANUARY
+
THANK YOU!
VEGAN OPTIONS
@HumaneLeagueUK
@WeAreVeganuary
VEGANUARY

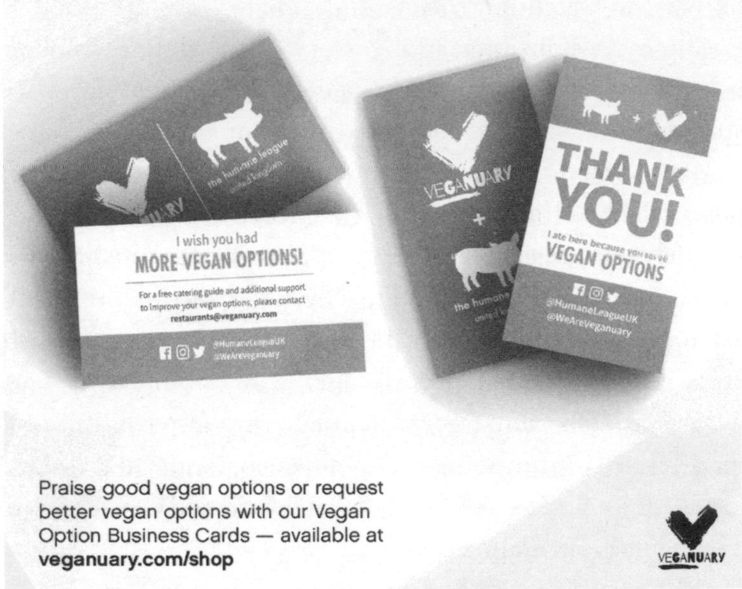

Praise good vegan options or request better vegan options with our Vegan Option Business Cards — available at **veganuary.com/shop**

INTERNATIONAL CUISINE

Plant-based eaters are usually well fed at restaurants that serve international dishes. From Chinese and Thai to Lebanese and North African, some delicious and common dishes may already be vegan, or can easily be adapted. When ordering, it's prudent to communicate your vegan needs clearly – as a rule of thumb, a vegetarian diet is well understood across cultures but the term vegan could cause confusion if communication is strained. Stating that you're a *strict vegetarian* and that you do not eat meat, fish, dairy and eggs can often be the best approach to take the stress out of ordering.

Here are some popular favourites and some handy hints on what to watch out for:

Chinese restaurants: spring rolls; bean curd (tofu) in black bean or Szechuan sauce; vegetable dishes, including bean-sprouts and sweet-and-sour; rice or rice noodles.

Watch out for: egg noodles (choose rice noodles instead, often called vermicelli); egg in fried rice; oyster sauce (there's a widely used vegan version made with oyster mushrooms, but some of them do contain real oyster extract – if in doubt, ask to see the bottle); dried shellfish (often used as a garnish on seaweed and other dishes).

Indian restaurants: vegetable samosas and pakoras; vegetable curries, from biryani to vindaloo; and side dishes, including lentil dhal and bhindi bhaji (okra). Add chapatis, rice, poppadums and chutneys.

Watch out for: yoghurt; ghee (clarified butter – sometimes used instead of oil); paneer (cheese); onion bhajis, which will usually contain egg (even though the store-bought versions can often be safe); naan breads which usually contain yoghurt.

Mexican restaurants: totopos (corn chips and tomato dip); guacamole; veggie tacos and tortillas; bean burritos; pozole (corn stew); vegetable or bean chilli; refried beans; potato skins.

Watch out for: cheese and sour cream.

Japanese restaurants: vegetarian gyoza (dumplings); tempura; miso soup; vegetable or avocado rolls; tofu dishes; ramen; vegetable curries.

Watch out for: ponzu sauce (contains tuna); surimi (fish

paste); mayonnaise and cream cheese (in westernised veggie sushi); Worcestershire sauce (sometimes called Bulldog sauce – contains anchovies and is used to flavour stews and soups).

Italian restaurants: Pasta pomodoro, arrabiata or Napoli; minestrone soup; vegetarian pizza without cheese; garlic bread (made with olive oil, not butter); olives; salads.

Watch out for: fresh egg pasta; parmesan (stop them before they sprinkle!)

Thai restaurants: Tofu or vegetable satay; tempura; soups and som tum salad; red, green or Masaman curries; stir-fried vegetables; coconut rice; noodles.

Watch out for: nam pla (fish sauce) – it can sneak its way into all Thai dishes (particularly curries) but, if the food is freshly prepared, they can leave it out at your request.

Lebanese restaurants: hummus; baba ghanoush (aubergine dip); tabbouleh; falafel; batata harra (spicy potatoes); fava bean dip; okra, beans or aubergines cooked in tomato sauce; flatbreads.

Watch out for: yoghurt; kashk (dairy); labneh (strained yoghurt cheese).

North African restaurants: harira soup; vegetable tagine; couscous; potatoes chermoula; flatbreads; salad.

Watch out for: honey; cheese; yoghurt.

> 'Through Veganuary, I learned about vegan products I could purchase at regular grocery stores, and also tips for eating out at non-vegan/vegetarian restaurants. After my first month, I was pleasantly surprised at how smooth my transition went. Veganuary was like my personal vegan mentor and I still rely on it for advice and information.'
>
> *Britt C., Kansas, US, Veganuary Class of 2017*

EATING AT FRIENDS' HOUSES

How do you break the news to your friends and family that the meals they have cooked for you before aren't going to go down so well on your next visit? You don't want to upset or offend, and nor do you want to be a massive pain in the backside. Besides, you can already hear the questions and jokes that are coming your way.

The great thing about trying vegan for a month is that it helps others around you accept the new diet, too. If you say that you're just trying it for a month to see how it feels, people will understand much more readily than if you just told them out of the blue that this former meat addict has gone vegan. That's when the questions will be fired at you in a rapid volley. But telling them that you're just trying it for a few weeks will probably elicit no more than an *OK*, shortly followed by *What will I feed you?*

It's usually a good idea to find out what your host is planning to cook on the occasion. You may be able to suggest some tweaks to their menu, such as roasting potatoes in oil rather than goose fat, or using dairy-free margarine instead of butter on garlic bread. Perhaps the dish they are planning can easily be made vegan, but if not, rather than watch them melt down in panic at cooking a whole other meal just for you, why not suggest you bring your own main, and match it as closely as possible to theirs? If they'll be eating lasagne or chilli or beef bourguignon, bring a spinach lasagne, a three-bean chilli or a mushroom and red wine casserole. By matching your meals, you won't feel like the odd one out, you will draw less attention to yourself and you'll show the other guests that a vegan meal doesn't have to be so very different from a non-vegan one.

It might be tempting to go ahead and create some mind-blowingly showy vegan dish, with indoor fireworks and sprinkled with gold dust. That would certainly showcase the creativity of veganism; but it might be better to save the theatricals for when you invite people to eat at your home. You don't want to upstage your host. OK, well maybe you do just a little bit, but we'd suggest you resist those urges.

If your host is happy to adapt a meal for you, you might like to offer to bring a dessert for everyone. This is usually the course where a non-vegan host runs out of steam, and you find yourself sitting in front of a fruit salad which, any way you dress it up, is a) just fruit and b) not a proper dessert (trust us on this, we're experts).

You'll find amazing recipes online for vegan sticky toffee pudding, treacle tart, chocolate torte, Key lime pie and many other popular desserts. By bringing your favourite vegan treat, you'll take some pressure off your host, add to your own vegan cookery repertoire and show off vegan food. You'll also be sure to get a great dessert!

What about Christmas, Thanksgiving, weddings and birthdays? The same advice applies: find out what's being made, suggest a few tweaks so you can enjoy as many of the dishes as possible and offer to bring anything else. If the food you make looks amazing, your host may just borrow your recipes for next time.

DEALING WITH FAMILY AND FRIENDS*

While telling family and friends that you're trying veganism for a few weeks may not provoke a huge reaction, for some new vegans it can lead to one of two outcomes. First, your loved ones might find this the most hilarious thing that has *ever* happened. You'll have to put up with some truly original witticisms about wimpy vegans and eating grass. We know. Hilarious.

* This advice can be extended to colleagues, school mates and that guy you bump into at the gym – all of whom are bound to have an opinion at some point!

But what is equally likely to happen is that you, as a fresh-faced new vegan, brimming with enthusiasm, will immediately start trying to persuade all your friends to join you in this plant-based adventure.

Let's take a look at both these scenarios, starting with your terrifically funny friends. If you think they're likely to make you the butt of a million jokes before they just accept you've decided to try vegan, you could try *not* telling them for a few weeks, so when they start up with the tired old clichés, you can respond: *That's old news. I've been vegan for ages and you didn't even notice.* That might just take the wind out of their sails.

But if it's just your turn to be the target of their banter, rising to it certainly won't make it go away. You'll just have to laugh along and take it on the chin. In time, they'll lose interest, especially if they see you eating some great food, and notice you're kicking their butts at the gym or out on the pitch. If the joking becomes unbearable, the unscrupulous might consider starting a racy rumour about someone else to deflect attention, or sacking these friends and getting some new ones. We don't advise these approaches. For better or worse, these are the people who have stood by you in hard times, and they are your friends for a reason. And there isn't much you can do to shake off family. Besides, in our experience, those that laugh loudest are often the most interested. Give them a little space to ask the questions they are probably bursting to know and see how many of them in time follow your lead. You might be surprised.

Now, let's look at the other possible outcome. You'll be feeling so great on your plant-based diet; you'll be sleeping better, looking better, full of energy and with a clear conscience. You may even be feeling a little smug about it all. That's OK. When we switch to a diet that is good news for animals, great for our health, helps feed the world and protects the planet, we can all get a little exuberant, even evangelical. A word to the wise: self-righteousness doesn't go down well, and nor does haranguing people about all the reasons why they are wrong to eat animal products.

If you don't like being lectured, or having your faults, inconsistencies and personality flaws pointed out, you can be sure that others feel the same. The people in your life will be much more responsive to the benefits of eating plant-based foods when you're calm and rational, not when you're parked outside their house with a banner and a megaphone. Hot-headed arguments rarely end in anyone changing their views.

What does work is being a great example, and a nice person. Some of what you've learned may now be so obvious to you that it's easy to forget there was ever a time when you didn't know it, but for your friends and family this is a lot to take in. And the things that horrify us most can be the hardest to accept. It's a difficult thing, after all, to accept that the diet we've always chosen has an impact on the world's hungriest or causes suffering to millions of animals. If you blame others for these things, the shutters will come down, and they will tell you where to go. Exactly as you would if they had done the same to you.

Patience is key. Even when people hear about all the reasons that being vegan is wonderful, they'll still worry about what they will eat. Inside, we might be screaming *WHAT ABOUT THE ANIMALS?* or *YOU ARE KILLING THE PLANET!* But we should never forget these legitimate concerns about missing out on favourite foods. If we're honest, it may well have been our first reaction, too. And people are just scared of change. That's normal, and OK. We were, too.

Very rarely is it one definable thing that makes someone go vegan. It may be that you read an article, saw a film, overheard some people talking on the train, looked up some information online, binged on cheese straws, saw an advert, tried soya milk, talked to some friends, saw a farming investigation in a newspaper, watched another film, read a book, went to a talk, joined a social media group, tried out your local veggie restaurant and only then decided to give it a go.

Of course, however tolerant you are, at times you will face negative attitudes – others may even set out to trip you up and it can be upsetting. Accusations of hypocrisy could be thrown at you for a whole host of reasons, from buying bottled water to taking a flight or even driving a car. It's a common misconception that your new vegan status should go hand in hand with shunning a catalogue of lifestyle choices. Your go-to response could be something like 'Being vegan reduces my impact on the planet significantly – but of course there are other ways I could improve.' Remain polite and humble.

And similarly, don't be made to feel guilty about your

pre-vegan choices – your wallet might still be leather and you may still wear your favourite woollen jumper – whilst dietary change can be immediate, you're not expected to rush out and replace all your worldly possessions. A good approach is to slowly replace your belongings with vegan versions as and when you need to – and you can explain that to the people who challenge you on this.

Your friends are still at the very beginning and the pieces may or may not fall into place for them. But if you're patient, happy to answer questions and refrain from lecturing, hectoring and blaming them, you may find they decide to join you. Cooking them great food is an excellent place to start – or maybe give them a copy of this book!

VEGAN TRAVELLING

You've become something of an expert on the range of vegan goodies that can be found in your local shops and restaurants, but what happens when you travel further afield? Depending on where your travels take you, things might be trickier. In some countries, meat is at the centre of every meal, and is also in the sauce, and mixed in with the vegetables too. So, it's wise to undertake a little research before you leave your home, to find out what the region's delicacies are and what they're made from. Search online for other vegans who have visited the area, as they might have discovered something that can really help you.

Of course, it's also possible that you will be surprised to find there are dozens of vegetarian or vegan restaurants at your chosen location, or at least a few where you can find vegan options. Vanilla-Bean.com and HappyCow.net are great places to find this out. Lots of people become vegan tourists, planning their holidays around the places with the most vegan restaurants, and there's no shame in that! Food is an important part of a holiday and, while there are many cities where you'll find exceptional vegan food within a fascinating location, these are some of the cities that crop up over and over as the vegans' favourites.

1. Berlin, Germany
2. Melbourne, Australia
3. Tel Aviv, Israel
4. Los Angeles, USA
5. Vancouver, Canada
6. Chennai, India
7. Brighton, UK
8. Taipei, Taiwan
9. Warsaw, Poland
10. Barcelona, Spain

As for accommodation, wherever you're going, check beforehand that the hotel or guesthouse can cater for you. Most hotels can offer a basic breakfast – fresh fruit, bread and jam, tea and coffee, cereals and plant-based milks. Others may be able to whip you up something else on request. But if they aren't able to provide a main meal and you're worried about finding suitable fare in local restaurants, again, ask for advice from one of the many vegan social media groups online. There may be someone who has been there or who lives there and has valuable insider knowledge.

In areas where vegan restaurants are hard to find, you'll still always find vegan ingredients, so if you're still drawing a blank, you may prefer to go self-catering.

Or maybe you'd like to take a complete break from cooking and instead be fully pampered, in which case check out the growing range of exclusively vegetarian and vegan hotels.

To throw yourself into the Vegan Traveller experience, it's best to learn (or at least carry with you) some basic phrases: *I'm vegan* and *I don't eat meat, fish, milk or eggs* are good places to start. The Vegan Society in the UK produces a Vegan Passport app, which offers useful phrases in 78 languages including Hausa, Igbo, Xhosa and Zulu, and images for where language still falls short. They also produce a hard-copy phrasebook you can pull out when needed.

Online translation services might also save the day, although they are not always 100 per cent reliable. We certainly *hope* there were no fried ravens in those Slovenian chocolate wafers we ate! And therein lies a valuable lesson. We are more likely to make a mistake when travelling than we are at home. We may be reading labels in another language, relying on translations or just hoping that the charades we are acting out can be understood. Most of us have eaten something we *think* is vegan but we can't be sure. It's not about perfection. It's about doing our best.

Nonetheless, it's a good idea to be prepared. There's nothing worse than trawling the streets with your stomach growling while you search for a vegan restaurant you know is there but can't find. Make sure you pack some snacks in your luggage to see you through any such grumpy periods. Cereal bars, dried fruits and nuts and a chocolate bar or two should be packed alongside your swim kit and sunscreen. Hopefully you'll bring them home again, but you'll be glad to know you have them as back-up.

NUTRITION IN A NUTSHELL

So, you want to try being vegan but there's someone in your life telling you it can't be good for you, that you'll get sick, be anaemic and protein-deficient, lose weight and probably expire before the week is out. It's nice that they worry, but they really shouldn't. You can get all the nutrients you need on a vegan diet – but you should be aware that with so many plant-based products out there, is it also possible to be a junk food vegan. As with any diet, it's essential you get enough of the right nutrients and limit the stuff we all know to be bad for us. Here are a few things to look out for.

PROTEIN

It's very hard to be protein-deficient, and yet this is the nutrient that people worry about most. This may be because of a common misconception that you have to consume meat to get enough protein. You don't! Just because there is protein in meat doesn't mean it doesn't exist anywhere else. In fact, vegans simply do what cows, pigs, sheep and chickens do: we go directly to the source. Green vegetables (the superstars are kale, broccoli, seaweed and peas), beans and pulses (lentils, lima, edamame, pinto and black), grains (rice, pasta, quinoa and bulgur) and nuts (Brazils, peanuts, cashews, almonds, pistachios, pine nuts and walnuts) are all excellent sources of protein.

Protein is needed for healthy enzymes, hormones and antibodies, and to build and repair muscles, but how much of it do we need? Guidelines vary depending on gender, age, activity levels and even where you live, since different countries' governments give different recommended intakes. But, as an example, we'll take a 30-year-old woman, not pregnant, who is active, engaging in one hour per day of walking or jogging, or 30 minutes of running. Her requirement is 47g of protein a day. For an active man of similar age, the requirement is 56g.

If she were to eat peanut butter on toast for breakfast, one hummus and falafel wrap and a shepherd's pie (made with soya mince) for dinner, she would easily exceed her required protein intake. And that's before she adds in the dairy-free milk she puts in her tea, some bread with her soup, the green vegetables with her dinner (there is 4g in a serving of broccoli and 5g in peas), or the soya milkshake, cereal bar or handful of nuts she has as a snack.

These are the protein levels in some everyday vegan meals:

BREAKFAST

Peanut butter on toast (2 pieces) 15g

Typical cereal with soya yoghurt and a handful of nuts 13g

Porridge/oatmeal with a sprinkle of almonds or seeds 12g

LUNCH

Three-bean salad wrap (2 wraps) 18g

Beans on toast (2 pieces) 17g

Hummus and falafel wrap (3 falafels, one wrap) 15g

DINNER

Tofu and vegetable stir-fry with brown rice 32g

Veggie sausages* (2), potato and peas 26g

Shepherd's pie, made with soya mince 20g

Other great protein-rich vegan foods to look out for are seitan, which has an incredible 30g of protein per serving, tempeh, quinoa and cashew or almond nut butters. But there is protein in almost all foods, including pasta, potatoes and vegetables, and so it's actually really hard to go short of it with a balanced vegan diet. Bodybuilders looking to increase their intake for significant muscle gain can choose one of the many vegan protein powders on the market, and incorporate it into their diets via protein shakes or balls.

If anyone suggests that plant-eaters can't be muscular and

* Not all veggie sausages have high protein levels; check the label.

powerful, ask them to think about where elephants, rhinos, hippos, mountain gorillas, oxen, water buffalo and bison get their protein from. The answer is, of course, plants. Just try telling a gorilla she's protein-deficient.

CALCIUM

In the same way that some people think protein and meat are synonymous, it's common to hear people conflate calcium with milk. We absolutely need calcium for strong bones (along with its super sidekick Vitamin D, which helps us to absorb it) – but we don't need to drink cows' milk to get it.

Most of the calcium in our bodies can be found in our bones, so if we don't consume enough of it our bodies will use up this store, and that can weaken our bones. The loss of too much calcium can lead to osteoporosis later in life, so it's important to ensure that we get a good supply.

You can boost your intake with beans (especially black turtle beans, kidney beans and soya beans), kale, collards, watercress, okra, broccoli, sweet potato and butternut squash. (Spinach has loads of calcium but it's poorly absorbed due to the oxalic acid in the leaves.) You can also snack on dried figs and almonds, and include some tofu in your meals.

If you're buying plant milks, look for brands that are fortified with calcium, and the same goes for yoghurts, too. There's no need to restrict yourself to health foods in the quest for calcium – even delicious vegan milkshakes are often calcium-rich.

As for Vitamin D, there's no better source than the sun, and 15 minutes of exposure a day during spring, summer and autumn should suffice so long as your face, hands and arms are exposed. But older or obese people, those who don't spend time outside, and those who live in northern latitudes or who have darker skin,[1] could be at greater risk of deficiency and may wish to look out for dairy-free margarines, breakfast cereals and breads that are fortified with it. You may also consider a supplement. This is wise for everyone, no matter their diet, because a lack of Vitamin D is surprisingly common, and can affect muscles and mood as well.[2]

While we're talking bone health, it's wise to avoid smoking, as this is a risk factor for osteoporosis. We should also do regular weight-bearing exercise, such as walking, running, dancing, playing tennis or football or lifting weights in the gym.

IRON

Iron is needed for healthy red blood cells to carry oxygen around the body. If we don't get enough, there's a risk of iron-deficiency anaemia. That could be the source of the outdated 'pale, tired vegetarian' myth. The truth is that iron-deficiency anaemia is commonplace across all diets, and particularly in women who menstruate. For this reason, the

bodies are able to make almost all the fatty acids we need. There are two, however, that we cannot make and therefore it's absolutely essential that we eat them. For this reason they are called 'essential' fatty acids. They're known as omega-3 and omega-6.

Deficiency is associated with kidney disease, heart disease, Alzheimer's, osteoarthritis, bowel disease and depression.[8] So, where can we get these essential acids?

Omega-6 can be found plentifully in leafy vegetables, seeds, nuts, grains and most vegetable oils. It is very easy to get sufficient omega-6 on a balanced diet – but this is where things start to get a little tricky. In all people, regardless of their diet, omega-6 acids compete with omega-3 acids for use in the body. So we need to pay attention and ensure we are eating sufficient omega-3 on a daily basis. Small amounts can be found in nuts, seeds, soya products, beans, vegetables and whole grains but the best sources of omega-3 are:

- Leafy vegetables, such as Brussels sprouts, kale, spinach and salad leaves
- Walnuts
- Rapeseed oil
- Ground flaxseed[9]
- Flaxseed oil
- Soybeans and tofu[10]
- Black lentils, also known as urad dal and mungo beans (not to be confused with mung beans)[11]

Ground flaxseed? Have you ever heard anything more stereotypically vegan in all your life?!

Don't despair. These ground-up seeds are quite common, and can be found in most supermarkets and health food shops. Add them to smoothies or muffin recipes or sprinkle them on your breakfast cereal and you won't even notice that you're getting a massive health boost. Eating a handful of walnuts as a snack will go a long way to ensuring you're getting enough omega-3 each day. And the cod will get to keep their livers.

If you're worried about getting enough omega-3, physician and author Dr Michael Greger recommends taking 250mg of pollutant-free long-chain omega-3s in the form of supplements, two or three times per week. These are obtained from algae – the same place that fish get their omega-3 from! Vegan versions of these supplements are widely available.

VITAMIN B12

This little vitamin can be quite elusive. One study revealed that one in 12 British women between the ages of 19 and 39 are deficient despite consuming the recommended intake[12] and deficiency can bring some pretty unpleasant symptoms. So let's all agree to get enough B12!

This vitamin is present in animal products, but it isn't made by the animals themselves; it's created by the bacteria that live inside them. Since vegans don't want to eat the animals – or their delicious bacteria – we can get B12 by instead eating yeast extracts, nutritional yeast flakes and breakfast cereals and plant-based milks that are fortified with it. Check the packaging to be sure your chosen brand contains B12. The more we spread out our intake, the less we need to consume, so try to eat three portions a day of B12-fortified foods.

It's not just vegans who need to keep an eye on their B12 intake. People who suffer from Crohn's or lupus, or who drink heavily, are at risk of being deficient. Since the risk of deficiency increases with age, the advice given in the US is for everyone over the age of 50 to take a daily B12 supplement regardless of their dietary choices.

This is advice we should all follow to be sure we are getting enough B12. Supplements can be taken in tablet form or in a spray and the recommended amount is 1.5 micrograms per day.[13] Most vegans take some form of supplement just to be sure.

GETTING IT RIGHT!

It's entirely possible to eat a nutritionally balanced vegan diet and thrive as a result. But it's also possible to get it wrong. If we live on fizzy drinks and chocolate, we might be vegan but we shouldn't expect to stay healthy for long. As a vegan, you are likely to be challenged about your diet by family and friends who show their concern by becoming nutritional experts. Learning about nutrition will help you be able to put their minds at rest; but most importantly, it will give you the best chance of staying healthy.

There is an app we recommend that can help you hit all your targets – Dr Greger's Daily Dozen is available for iPhone and Android, and lets you track quite easily the foods you should aim to eat every day. Alternatively, you can download and print out the Daily Dozen wall chart from veganuary.com. If you're in any doubt, or have additional health conditions, always consult a medical professional.

VEGAN MYTHS

There are a lot of myths surrounding veganism and you're likely to be faced with at least one of them during your first few weeks as a vegan. Some myths, like *You won't get enough protein,* are so common that we can pretty much predict them. You can even play Vegan Myth Bingo and see how many you are confronted with (see page 135). Here are the most likely, and all the information you'll need to bat them away. Politely, of course.

1. What's the point? One person won't make a difference.

Au contraire. One person makes a very real difference!

The average British meat-eater consumes more than 11,000 animals in their lifetime[1], and many more animals are killed in the dairy and egg industries. By choosing to stop today, *a lot* of lives will be spared. It won't save the animals who are in farms and slaughterhouses right now, of course, but it is a simple rule of economics that when demand decreases, so does supply. As people buy fewer animal products, supermarkets and butchers will reduce their orders, and so fewer animals will be bred and killed. A growing number of farmers are already changing from farming cows to growing crops!

Not only are we sparing the lives of animals, we're shrinking our food-related carbon emissions by half.[2] These are no small things; and our impact is magnified still further because we are not going vegan all by ourselves. There are millions of us choosing to eat only animal-free foods and each of us influences others to enjoy meat-free meals, too. In fact, more than half of the people who take part in Veganuary say they have inspired someone else to go vegan. And if those people influence someone else too . . . you see what we mean?

What we achieve alone is something extraordinary to be proud of. Together, we are changing the whole world for the better, and every person's contribution counts.

2. Animals on high welfare farms have a good life and a humane death

The majority of farmed animals are reared intensively. If the package on the shelf doesn't specifically say 'free range' or 'organic' then the animal was almost certainly factory-farmed, and there is no point trying to kid ourselves that those chicken nuggets came from birds who spent their days roaming free. Even where we do make the effort to choose higher welfare meat, the reality for those animals may be very different to what we imagine. We may think of free range hens roaming in a pasture, pigs grubbing in a woodland or goats running around an expansive hillside. In most cases, this comforting vision is a long way from reality.

Free range hens do not live outdoors but instead are given access to it for a period of the day, if the weather permits. Since flock sizes are enormous and hens are territorial, many birds won't cross another's territory to get to the exit holes and they'll instead spend their entire lives inside a shed. And what of the outdoor space itself? Often, it's little more than a patch of dirt, and almost certainly not what is printed on the box, shown on the website, or the image you have in your mind.

Male chicks born into the free range egg industry will be gassed, crushed or minced alive on their first day of life because they are deemed useless. And when the females' productivity declines, being free range or organic won't save them from the slaughterhouse.

The vast majority of chickens reared for their meat are kept inside factory farms. Those who are reared under 'high welfare' schemes fare little better. For many, the painful joint problems that are endemic in the modern high yielding breeds mean their lives are miserable no matter what system they are reared in. When they are just a few weeks old, they are caught by their legs or necks, rammed into crates and trucked to the slaughterhouse.

For other animals, like pigs, free range usually means a patch of dirt and a metal arc. Pigs love to root, run and play. They like to socialise, build nests and explore; but none of this is afforded them on most commercial 'high welfare' farms.

There is no humane way to produce commercial quantities of milk. Cows, goats and sheep must be made pregnant and the offspring are often no more than unwanted by-products. Calves may go for veal production or be shot at birth. Cows who have their young taken away can bellow for them for days.

In some countries, cows are able to live outdoors all year round but in most parts of the world, even under 'high welfare' schemes, they are permitted out for just six months a year. Rather than making them stand out in the mud as the rain lashes down for the other half of the year, they are forced to stand around in their own faeces inside a barn. It's not clear which is preferable.

All animals – whether free range, organic, barn-reared, outdoor-bred or caged – end their lives in the same place. Investigations all around the world show that animals are terrified when they enter the slaughterhouse, and that those who were reared under 'high welfare' schemes in the UK were treated no better than those reared on factory farms.

3. You won't get enough protein

Oh dear. The person who tells you this has not yet worked out that meat and protein are not the same thing, nor have they realised that protein is found in almost everything we eat. A third misconception is how much protein we need. In Western Europe and the US, protein consumption is significantly higher than the recommended intakes[3] and this could be linked to health problems too,[4] so eating the right amount of protein, from the right sources, is key.

Protein is made from amino acids, some of which our bodies make while others must come from food. Eating a variety of cereals, beans, nuts and vegetables can provide all the amino acids our bodies require[5] but if there is a small voice nagging away inside your brain, telling you that this cannot be so and that as a vegan your muscles will inevitably atrophy, visit www.plantbuilt.com and www.greatveganathletes.com, and check out the physiques of the vegan bodybuilders, weightlifters and powerlifters. Look on in awe.

Meat is not the only source of protein but if the doubters still doubt you, ask them this: where does an elephant or bison get his or her protein from? The answer, of course, is plants.

For more information on protein requirements, see page 107.

4. It's natural to eat meat

What is 'natural'? The chicken who cannot live more than six weeks, the turkey who can't even breed without human help or the cow selectively bred to produce far more milk than is good for her health?

Farmed animals are artificially inseminated, endure many mutilations and are selectively bred to have large litters. They're engineered to put on weight fast, unless they're an egg-laying hen, in which case they're bred *not* to put on weight, as that would be a waste of food. They are fed artificial feed, have their breeding cycles manipulated with hormone sponges inserted into their vaginas[6] and the length of their day is managed through artificial lighting. It's not possible to imagine anything less natural than the animal farming industry.

Often what people mean by this is: *Haven't we always done it?* And *Don't we have all the right biological equipment to eat meat?* And the answers to those questions are *no* and *not really*.

The food our ancestors ate would have depended on what era they lived in and where in the world, as well as the season, the climate and the weather, so we can't make any generalisations about what we have 'always eaten'.

We do know that humans were predominantly gatherers like other apes, only scavenging meat that true carnivores left behind. Take a look at our hands and teeth, which are useless for ripping flesh, and our lack of speed, which would see even a lame antelope outrun us. These things are not a problem for true carnivores, like jaguars and tigers. The canine teeth people cite as 'proof' that we should eat meat look nothing like the canines of carnivores and are misnamed.

Obviously, we can tolerate a bit of meat in our diet, but our bodies have never really adapted to it. Our intestines are long, and look more like those belonging to our herbivorous friends than to our carnivorous ones. Carnivores have short intestines as they need to move meat out of their system quickly before it putrefies and kills them. Food poisoning in people is still predominantly caused by animal products and meat continues to harm the human body in many other ways, including through higher rates of heart disease, some cancers and diabetes.

5. You'll feel weak or ill

Vegan food is nutritious and the vast majority of people who take part in Veganuary say they feel better as a result of going without animal products. Even within the first few weeks, they report that they have more energy, have lost weight and sleep better. Many also say they have improved digestion, sleep, skin, hair and nails.

For most people, switching to a vegan diet feels great in the short term, but crucially it also reduces their risks over the long term from diseases like cancer, heart disease and diabetes.

If someone becomes ill when they switch to a vegan diet, then generally one of two things is happening: either they have caught a bug or developed a condition and would have become ill anyway, or they are eating all the wrong foods.

It's entirely possible to be a junk food vegan these days, with so many convenience foods out there. If you fail to eat good, wholesome, nutritious foods, you're more likely to feel under the weather, and that's true whatever your diet. If a person chooses to live off biscuits and crisps, you can't really blame their deficiencies on veganism. It's their food choices that are the problem. Conversely, if they eat a balanced diet (check out the section on nutrition) then they're very unlikely to become ill as a result.

All the nutrients you need can be found in a well-planned vegan diet. So if you find you're falling short of, say, enough iron, then make sure you include plenty of whole grains, beans, peas, nut butters and green leafy vegetables in your diet.

We should realise, too, that it takes a little time for a good diet to undo the damage of a poor one. Online nutrition trackers and apps can be useful in giving you a rough idea about whether you are consistently failing to get enough of a particular nutrient. If this is the case, you'll need to adjust your diet to account for it, but the good news is that this can all be done on a vegan diet, and there's no need to go back to the animal products that can cause so much sickness in the long run.

It may take a little time to adapt and get into the groove of a vegan diet, and you may notice some changes to your body in that time – including in your weight, skin and frequency of bathroom visits – but if you start to experience unpleasant symptoms, don't make assumptions about the cause. Instead see a doctor for advice.

6. I'm sporty so veganism won't suit me

Formula One driver Lewis Hamilton is vegan, as is heavyweight boxer David Haye. World champion tennis player Novak Djokovic is so taken with plant-based foods that he has opened his own vegan restaurant, while tennis champions Serena and Venus Williams also tout the benefits of eating plant-based while in training.

American footballers Griff Whalen and David Carter are vegan. David is known as the 300-lb vegan and eats 10,000 calories a day to maintain his extraordinary fitness regime. If you think eating vegan will make you weak, think again. Patrik Baboumian is an Iranian-born German strongman – Germany's Strongest Man, in fact – who has set four world records in various strength disciplines and can bench-press 463lb and deadlift 794lb. He says: 'My strength needs no victims.' And he's not alone. There are many more strength athletes who are vegan, including Olympian weightlifter Kendrick Farris.

Do you like a little more contact in your sport but worry that going vegan will somehow make you soft? We dare you to put that proposition to mixed martial art champion Mac Danzig, European jiu-jitsu champion Emilia Tuukkanen or Austrian champion boxer Melanie Fraunschiel. All 100 per cent vegan, all 100 per cent badass.

> 'Rugby is a high-collision contact sport so no matter what you eat or what you do, you're going to be sore from the knocks and the bruises. But since going vegan I can't really remember the last time I had delayed onset muscle soreness. And that obviously helps me give more to the next training session.'
>
> *Anthony Mullally, professional rugby league player, UK*

As for runners, you'd be hard-pressed to keep pace with Scott Jurek, Rich Roll and Fiona Oakes. Scott has won the Western States 100-mile endurance race no fewer than seven times. He won the Miwok 100k three times, the 246k Spartathlon race twice, the Leona Divide 50k race four times and has set ten ultramarathon records. Rich has competed in the world's top tier of Ironman events and pushed his body beyond extremes when he completed five Ironman-distance triathlons in under a week. His story is made all the more astonishing as he only started to train at the age of 40, when he also adopted a plant-based diet. Fiona is an amateur marathon runner who holds three world records, has come in the top 10 in several international marathons and in the top 20 in both London and Berlin. Oh, and remember Carl Lewis? Yep – he was vegan too.

Team GB triathlete Dan Geisler took a silver medal at the World Championships eight months after going vegan. He described his move to a plant-based diet as 'a very, very good decision'.

Ireland rugby league international Anthony Mullally went vegan and reported more energy, better recovery and no loss of strength, which all contributed to him having the most consistent season of his career. World Champion figure skater Meagan Duhamel, international rugby union player and cyclist Johanna Jahnke and free running champion Tim Shieff are vegan, too, showing that no matter what your sport, you can thrive, take titles and smash records on a vegan diet.

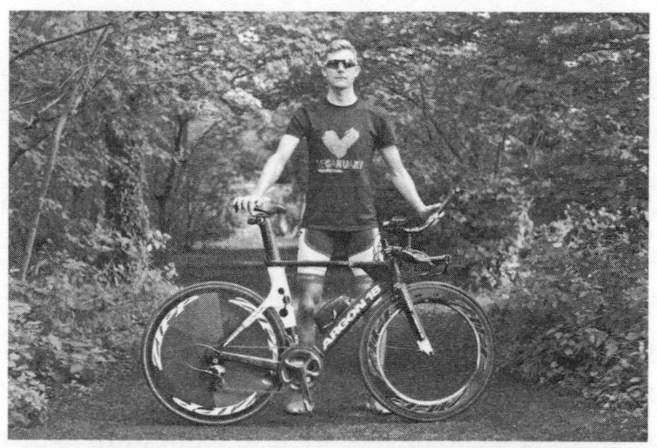

Team GB triathlete Dan Geisler.

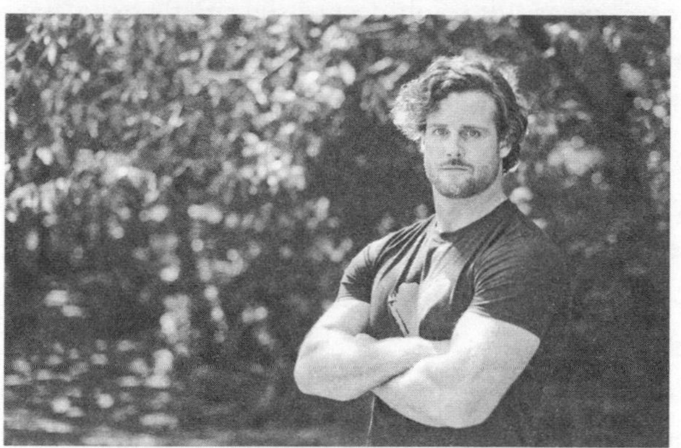

Ireland rugby league international Anthony Mullally.

7. We need meat to be healthy

Quite the opposite. A plant-based diet cuts the risk of developing heart disease, type 2 diabetes and some kinds of cancers. Vegans typically have lower cholesterol levels, lower blood pressure and a healthier Body Mass Index than meat-eaters. And those who choose plant proteins over animal proteins live longer, too.[7]

Processed red meat has now been classified as a Group 1 carcinogen,[8] putting it in the same category as smoking and asbestos. Meat is said to be 'processed' if it has undergone salting, curing, smoking, fermentation or any other process to enhance its flavour or improve its preservation. This includes bacon, hot dogs, ham, sausages, salami, corned beef, biltong, beef jerky, canned meat and meat-based sauces. The evidence is clear: these processed red meats can cause bowel cancer; and there's some evidence that connects them to stomach and pancreatic cancers, too.[9]

Unprocessed red meat has been classified as Group 2A, which means it is 'probably carcinogenic to humans'[10]. There are clear associations between eating red meat and developing bowel cancer,[11] and there is also evidence of links to prostate cancer.[12]

While some people think that switching to white meat is the answer, the US-based non-profit organisation Physicians Committee for Responsible Medicine says we should think again: 'faeces, toxic chemicals, superbugs, carcinogens, and cholesterol are likely hiding in every bite'.[13] In the UK, three-quarters of chicken carcasses are contaminated with campylobacter, which can cause diarrhoea, cramping, abdominal pains, vomiting and fever. More than a quarter of a million people a year are made sick by the bug, and 100 people die.[14] In Canada, there are 145,000 illnesses from this bug each year[15] and in the US, it is thought to affect more than 1.3 million people a year.[16]

Salmonella is another nasty bug that proliferates in chicken meat, as well as in eggs and unpasteurised milk. In the US, it causes one million foodborne illnesses and kills 380 people each year.[17] In Canada, 88,000 people a year are infected with it,[18] with children and the elderly particularly vulnerable. Why take the risk?

8. It's impossible to give up cheese

Often when someone is struggling to become vegan, cheese is the thing that holds them back. It's almost as if that stuff was addictive! In fact, researchers have found that the casein in cheese can trigger the brain's opioid receptors, which produces a feeling of euphoria. This may explain in part why cheese often seems to be the thing that new vegans miss the most.

But cheese is not addictive like drugs are addictive. Anyone can give it up, although we know it can take some mighty willpower, at least to begin with.

If you really want to break that cheese habit, there are things you can do to make it a little bit easier: avoid the cheese aisle in your local supermarket (why risk the temptation?), go to pizza restaurants where they offer dairy-free cheese; and try out the range of plant-based cheeses available in shops now. Don't restrict yourself to what's available in your local shops; there are many more you can order online, and you'll be sure to find some that suit your tastes. Of course, they won't taste exactly like dairy cheese because they're not dairy cheese – and no two dairy cheeses taste the same anyway. But some vegan cheeses taste *really* good, so pile up the crackers and pickles and have your very own vegan cheese taster session to find out which are the ones for you.

If you steer clear of dairy cheese for 31 days, something unexpected might well happen to you. Lots of vegans report that, where once they would push their noses up against the cheese counter, trying to inhale it even if they'd decided against eating it, very quickly once going vegan the smell of cheese becomes less appealing. Unpleasant, even. Rancid and sweaty-sock-ish.

Our taste buds also change very quickly, and once the habit is broken, you may find that you're completely turned off by the very thing that you once missed so much.

9. Isn't soya destroying our planet?

Large expanses of land are needed to grow the quantity of soya beans the world requires, and swathes of ancient forests and savannah have been felled as a result.[19] Deforestation is devastating for biodiversity and these ancient ecosystems, once felled, are lost for ever.

It's easy to blame the people who eat tofu or drink soya

milk because they're the most visible consumers of these beans. But they are not the *main* consumers of soya. Most of the world's crop, in fact, is fed to farmed animals, including to fish.[20] Most of the world's soya is indirectly eaten by meat-eaters.

We have to acknowledge that all farming has an impact on the environment, and that the land we use to grow any food may be less diverse and sustain fewer species than had it been left in a wild state. But the advice given by the World Wild Fund for Nature for reducing the amount of soya grown is to limit consumption of animal products and, in particular, meat.[21]

Vegans who have an allergy to soya find it's perfectly possible to get sufficient protein from other plant sources, so it is not essential that a plant-based diet include this bean. But soya itself isn't the problem. Trying to grow enough soya to feed billions of farmed animals is.

10. The desert island myth

This is less of a myth and more of a question: *If you were stranded on a desert island, would you eat meat then?*

We need to be straight with you. You're no more likely to be stranded on a desert island after going vegan than you were before, but you will be asked about it so often that there may be times when you wish you were stranded far, far away.

Since there is unlikely to be a delicatessen on this island, the question isn't so much *Would you eat meat?* as *Would you kill an animal?* We can overlook for now how these animals came to be on the island, and we could answer simply that, however they got there, they appear to be thriving, so we'll just eat what they're eating. It is a lot safer to eat nuts, roots, tubers and berries than to hunt down wild beasts with a stick. (We're assuming we didn't get washed up with a loaded gun, a set of butchery knives, *Evisceration for Dummies* and a camping stove.)

Animals don't walk over and lie down for you, you know. You'd have to track them, surprise them, overpower them and cut their throats. In this struggle, there's a decent chance that you'll be the one who ends up as someone's dinner. No offence. It's just that they're a wild animal and have spent their whole life successfully not getting eaten and you're, you know, an accountant or a teacher or a bus driver.

The savvy will have spotted that this question is not really about desert islands, it's about finding the limit to your resolve and principles. *Would you really rather starve to death than eat an animal?* This question can be flipped on the questioner: *If you were living on an island with loads of wholesome plant-based foods, would you still choose to eat the corpses of tortured animals?*

Failing that approach, you can usually stop the conversation with: *If I was hungry enough, I would eat you.*

VEGAN MYTH BINGO

A plant-based diet is great for people, animals and the planet. But some tired myths linger on. Tell enough people you're vegan and there's a good chance that you will be treated to one or more of these gems. It's not their fault, they don't know any better!

So come join us and play vegan myth bingo. First one to ten gets a carrot!

WHERE DO YOU GET YOUR PROTEIN?	BUT, CHEESE THOUGH...?	PLANTS FEEL PAIN
VEGANS ARE WEAK	EATING MEAT IS A PERSONAL CHOICE	IF WE DIDN'T EAT ANIMALS THEY'D TAKE OVER
ONE PERSON WON'T MAKE A DIFFERENCE	IT'S NATURAL TO EAT MEAT	IT'S TOO EXPENSIVE

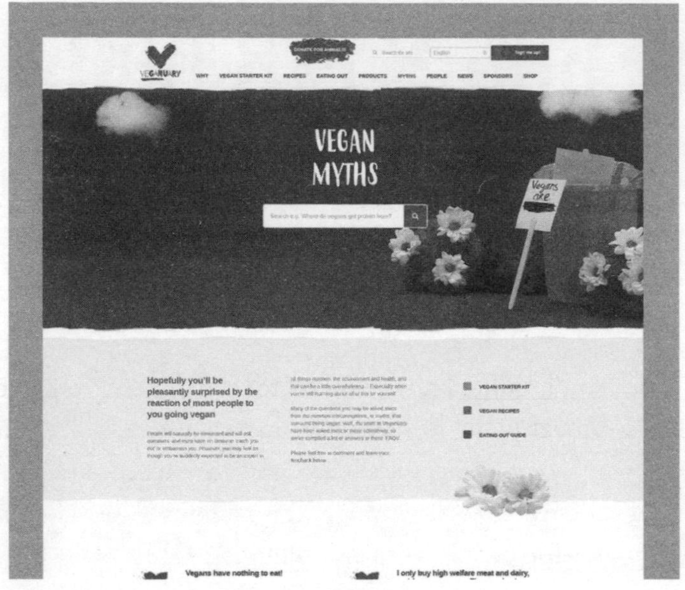

Found a myth that we've not mentioned? Check out the myths section at veganuary.com for all the responses you'll ever need.

MEAL PLANS

If you don't quite know where to start, we've created a series of meal plans to help you, and they can all be found at veganuary.com. There are quick and easy plans and family-friendly plans, as well as plans for athletes, those avoiding gluten and for people with nut allergies.

> 'Definitely do it. There's no down side to signing up for Veganuary. You can participate to the extent that you want – just read and ponder the daily emails, which contain recipes, info about some of the issues and inspiring stories; or go ahead and try some of the recipes; or decide to have 'meat-free Monday' each week; or dive in and commit to eating no animal products at all for the month.'
>
> *Heather K., Victoria, Australia,*
> *Veganuary Class of 2017*

Below are two meal plans. The first is for your first week transitioning to a vegan diet, and the second for when you're feeling a bit more adventurous. You'll find the underlined recipes at veganuary.com.

MEAL PLAN 1

Getting started: keeping it simple

Monday

BREAKFAST

Porridge/oatmeal with bananas and seeds, made with a plant milk of your choice – remember some come sweetened, some don't.

LUNCH

Falafel, rocket (arugula) and sweet chilli sauce sandwich

DINNER

Shepherd's pie, using soya mince or lentils instead of meat. Remember dairy-free margarine and milk for the mashed potato!

Tuesday

BREAKFAST

Breakfast cereal of your choice with dairy-free yoghurt

LUNCH

Vegetable soup (either bought or home-made using vegetable stock) with crusty bread

DINNER

Fajitas. Use vegan meat strips or strips of seitan or tofu. Or try the portobello fajitas on veganuary.com. Serve with guacamole and salsa

Wednesday

BREAKFAST

Avocado and tomatoes on toast

LUNCH

Couscous salad, made with peppers, herbs, chickpeas (garbanzo), salad onions, cucumber, tomatoes and anything else you like. Add vinaigrette dressing or egg-free mayo

DINNER

Pasta with tomato sauce (home-made or shop-bought) with a green salad and garlic bread

Thursday

BREAKFAST

Fruit smoothie and wholemeal toast with your choice of peanut butter, yeast extract or jam

LUNCH

Veggie sausage sandwich with mustard or ketchup

DINNER

Courgette and sun-dried tomato risotto. Serve with asparagus, broccoli or a mixed salad

Friday

BREAKFAST

Super-healthy, superfood yoghurt – your choice of dairy-free yoghurt with berries, fruit, nuts and seeds

LUNCH

Hummus and salad wraps – choose your flavour of hummus and your favourite veg

DINNER

Pizza – either a shop-bought vegan pizza (you may need to order online) or buy the dough base, and add tomato sauce, your choice of toppings and dairy-free cheese

Saturday

BREAKFAST

Maple cinnamon granola

LUNCH

Roasted red pepper soup with cheese on toast

DINNER

Sausages and mash. Your choice of vegan sausages, with mashed potatoes, peas and gravy

Sunday

BREAKFAST

The full fried breakfast: choose from vegan sausages and vegan bacon, tofu scramble, grilled tomatoes, fried mushrooms, baked beans and toast or veggie bread

LUNCH

Ginger, coconut and lemongrass soup

DINNER

Roast dinner. All your favourite roast potatoes, parsnips, carrots and celeriac with a centrepiece of your choice. Why not try 'chicken' and leek pie, smoky veggie wellington or a tomato and mushroom roast?

MEAL PLAN 2

Going Gourmet: OK, let's do this vegan thing

Monday

BREAKFAST

Peanut butter and banana smoothie

LUNCH

Speedy sweet potato quesadillas with salad

DINNER

Red tofu curry with rice (or quinoa)

Tuesday

BREAKFAST

Choc and raspberry porridge

LUNCH

Vegan quiche served with a Waldorf salad

DINNER

Beetroot and kale burgers with balsamic red onions

Wednesday

BREAKFAST

Banana pancakes with blueberries and maple syrup

LUNCH

Portobello mushrooms and tofu scramble ciabatta sandwich

DINNER

Black bean chilli with rice and a green salad

Thursday

BREAKFAST

Apple cinnamon wholemeal waffles

LUNCH

Chilli tomato and basil baked beans on toast

DINNER

One-pot linguine with olives, capers and sun-dried tomatoes

Friday

BREAKFAST

Breakfast burritos

LUNCH

Refried beans with corn tortillas

DINNER

BBQ pulled jackfruit with corn tacos

Saturday

BREAKFAST

Toast with garlicky butterbean toast topper

LUNCH

Asparagus with white miso and mint dressing, served with summer couscous

DINNER

Turkish tofu and spinach börek

Sunday

BREAKFAST

Tortilla española

LUNCH

Leek latkes with cauliflower cheese

DINNER

Vegetable coulibiac with porcini mushroom sauce

SNACKS:

Fresh fruit, dried fruit, crackers, crisps, dairy-free chocolate, cereal bars and mixed nuts. For the weekend, why not make cookies, spiced plum muffins or brownies?

DRINKS:

Fruit juice, coffee, tea, herbal tea, water, squash – whatever you normally have

DESSERTS:

Choose from the many delicious desserts on veganuary.com, including cakes, cheesecakes and truffles. There are some healthier options, too!

RECIPES TO GET YOU STARTED!

> 'I'd tried to be a vegetarian a number of times over the years but always slipped back. I guess with Veganuary I thought that, at best, I'd learn a few recipes to add to weekly meals. I never imagined that over the course of the month I'd take on a full vegan diet!'
>
> *Melanie R., Lennoxtown, Scotland,*
> *Veganuary Class of 2017*

Breakfast: Maple Cinnamon Granola

(SERVES 2–4)

INGREDIENTS

3 cups rolled oats

½ cup almonds, roughly chopped

½ cup pumpkin seeds
½ cup sunflower seeds
2 tsp ground cinnamon
2 tbsp almond butter
3 tbsp maple syrup

INSTRUCTIONS

- Heat the oven to 180°C.
- In a bowl, mix together the dry ingredients. Set aside.
- In a saucepan, melt the almond butter and maple syrup over a low heat, then stir it through the oaty mixture.
- Line a baking tray with greaseproof paper and pour in the mixture. Pat down roughly.
- Cook for 20 minutes, then leave to cool in the tray. Store the granola in an airtight container.

Lunch: Ginger, Coconut and Lemongrass Soup

(SERVES 2–4)

INGREDIENTS

1 tsp coconut oil
1 onion, diced
½ bunch spring onions, diced
4 cloves garlic, minced
1 stalk lemongrass, left whole but crushed with the flat of a knife

1 thumb-sized piece fresh ginger, peeled and finely diced
2 carrots, peeled and chopped into coins
3 cups water
1 can coconut milk, full fat
¼ cup tamari
2 tbsp vegetable stock
2 red bell peppers, sliced
10 mushrooms, sliced
Salt and pepper to taste
Lime, spring onion or coriander for garnish

INSTRUCTIONS

- Heat the coconut oil in a pan over a medium heat. Add the onion, spring onion and garlic and cook for a minute.
- Add the lemongrass, ginger and carrots and cook until soft.
- Add the water, coconut milk, tamari and vegetable stock, and bring to the boil, then add the red peppers and mushrooms.
- Reduce the heat and simmer for 15–20 minutes.
- Remove the lemongrass stalk before serving, and season to taste.
- Serve with a wedge of lime, diced spring onion or roughly chopped coriander.

Dinner: One-Pot Linguine with Olives, Capers and Sun-dried Tomatoes

(SERVES 2)

INGREDIENTS

200g dried linguine (or spaghetti)
500g passata with onion and garlic
250ml water
1 red chilli, deseeded and finely sliced
6 pieces sun-dried tomato (that have been preserved in oil), chopped
50g pitted black olives, halved
1 tbsp capers
1 tsp sugar
2 tbsp olive oil
Handful fresh basil, roughly chopped

INSTRUCTIONS

- Place the linguine flat into the bottom of a large, lidded saucepan. You may need to break it in half to make it fit.
- Cover the linguine with the passata, and add the water. Bring to the boil and reduce to a simmer, stirring to ensure the pasta does not stick to the bottom of the pan as it softens.
- Add the chilli, sun-dried tomato, olives, capers, sugar and olive oil. Stir well and cover.
- Cook on a medium heat for 10–11 minutes, stirring regularly, until the pasta is cooked through.

- Stir in the basil, and serve.

Sweet Snack: Chocolate Chip Brownies

(MAKES 6–8 BROWNIES)

INGREDIENTS

½ cup plain flour
½ cup wholewheat flour
½ cup cocoa powder
2 tbsp cornstarch
1 tsp baking powder
¼ tsp salt
½ cup granulated sugar
¼ cup cane sugar, blended into a powder
¼ cup vegetable oil
¼ cup maple syrup
¼ cup any non-dairy milk
2 tsp vanilla extract
¼ cup vegan dark chocolate chips
⅓ cup walnuts, coarsely chopped

INSTRUCTIONS

- Heat the oven to 180°C, and put an 8 x 8-inch (20 x 20cm) pan lined with greaseproof paper into the oven.
- Sift together the plain flour, wholewheat flour, cocoa powder, cornstarch, baking powder and salt. Add the granulated sugar and cane sugar.

- In a separate bowl, mix together the oil, maple syrup, non-dairy milk and vanilla extract. Whisk.
- Pour the wet ingredients into the dry ingredients, and mix until smooth. Set aside for 10 minutes.
- Stir in the chocolate chips and nuts, then spoon the mixture into the heated pan, and spread into an even layer.
- Bake for 20–25 minutes, until the top is set and dry and the sides have pulled away just slightly from the pan. If a skewer comes out clean, they are cooked.
- Cool to room temperature if you can wait that long. Or serve immediately with dairy-free vanilla ice cream.

VEGAN
RECIPES
Discover fresh and
exciting vegan food
Delicious vegan recipes
from all over the world

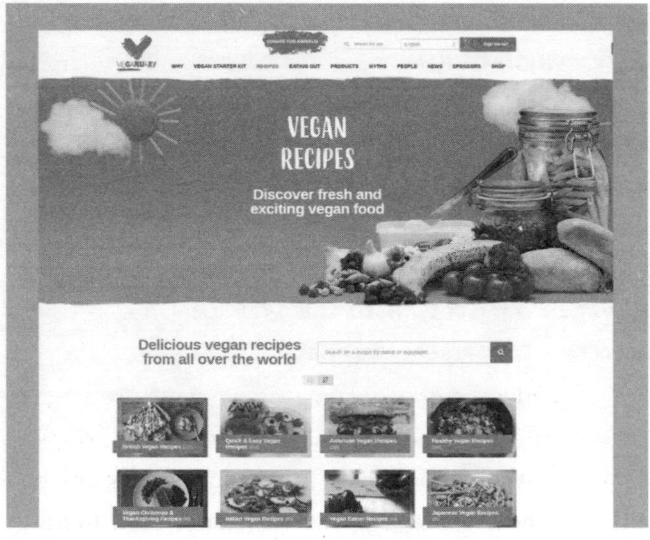

The Veganuary website has hundreds of tasty recipes.

THE BIG QUESTIONS

For new vegans and those just dipping their toes into the plant-based pool, there are inevitably a lot of questions that crop up. The Veganuary website and our social media platforms are great places to start searching for additional advice and information, but there are a few questions that may still linger in your mind, and not everyone feels able to voice these aloud. We hear you, and we hope this section helps.

WHAT IF I MESS UP?

So, you've pledged to try vegan for 31 days. You're armed with as much info as your head can hold and you've read every label in the supermarket. Your cupboards are packed with plant-based foods and you've calculated how many steps lie between you and your nearest vegan burrito. You've registered to take part in Veganuary, which you can do at any time of year if you don't want to wait until January, and those support emails will be arriving in your inbox any moment. You are on your vegan way. But still you worry, *What if I mess up?*

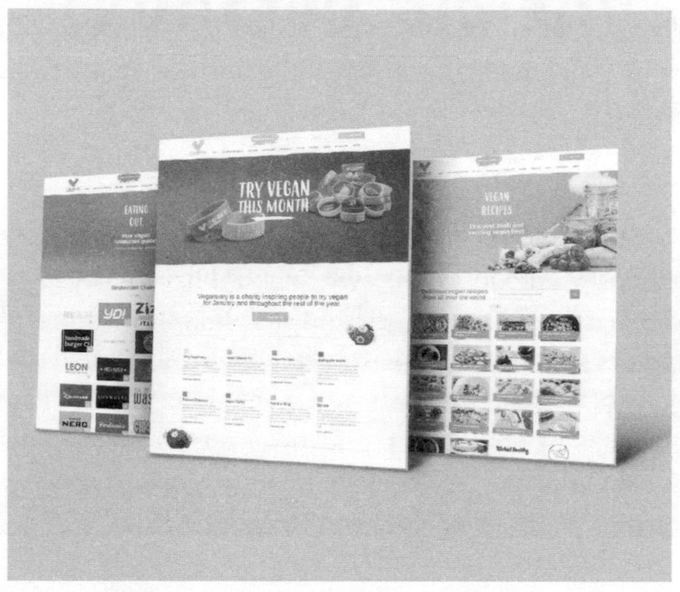

The Veganuary website is packed with useful information.

There is no messing up. Taking part in Veganuary signals that you're going to give plant-based eating a good go for those 31 days, but there is no one hiding in your fridge to leap out at you if you come home with a cheese-encrusted pizza late one night. You won't be shamed on social media or outed on the national news.

If you make a mistake or have a slip-up, it's OK. These

things happen, and we've been there. Old habits don't always let go of us, even if we're trying our hardest to shake them off. And even the best-intentioned resolve can weaken after a drink or two. Our advice is: don't let it set you back. If you really want to stick with trying vegan, put the lapse to the back of your mind. You just made a mistake, so start again tomorrow.

> 'I just wanted to say that this has been the most supportive group I have ever joined! I have enjoyed Veganuary, one or two slip-ups, but I am learning to forgive myself. I have loved the way we have shared and discussed options.'
>
> *Rachel J., Stockport, UK,*
> *Veganuary Class of 2017*

I'M STRUGGLING! WHAT SHOULD I DO?

No one is underestimating how difficult it is to change life-long food habits, especially when those around you are continuing to eat what they've always done. Nights out, meals with friends and special occasions can all take some getting used to, and for some people, trying vegan can feel like a lonely experience. And when all you can think about is your cravings for cheese, it's hard to remember why you ever thought trying vegan was a good idea. If you know deep down that you'd like to try vegan but you're struggling to stick with it, these top tips might just get you through.

- Remind yourself why you're doing this! Write down all the reasons why you wanted to give veganism a try, and see if they remain. Re-read the *Why Try Vegan?* section of this book, and check out the books and films we recommend on pages 158–60.

- Connect with other vegans by joining vegan groups in real life or online. The Veganuary Facebook page is full of supportive vegans – some of them are new and still adjusting to this way of life, while others are vegan veterans. Don't be afraid to voice your concerns or ask for some moral support. Vegans are, by and large, a caring, compassionate group of people who know how to pick you up, make you laugh and give you that support when you need it most. For young vegans, www.TeenVgn.com is a great community.

- Read the testimonials within this book. They're inspirational, and written by people who have experienced exactly what you're experiencing, and have got through it.

- Remember it's OK to take it slow. It may be better to replace one product at a time and transition over a period than to leap straight in if you're finding it difficult. If there's one thing you think you'll miss most of all, leave that until last – but ask your new vegan friends what alternatives are out there.

- Keep a diary so you can remind yourself how far you've come and what you've already achieved, how amazing you felt on the good days, the new favourite foods that you've discovered and why this is important to you.

- Be good to yourself. Being vegan isn't about deprivation! Treat yourself with a bar of chocolate (not just the dark ones; there are lots of vegan 'milk' chocolates available, too!), a glass of wine or a meal out at your favourite vegan cafe or restaurant.

- Do what you love! If you love to cook, treat yourself to a great vegan cookbook and test out some new recipes. If you're a runner, join the Vegan Runners – they meet in real life as well as online. Try to make your vegan journey a joyful experience.

- Visit a vegan festival – there are lots of them springing up all over the world, and as you jostle with hundreds or thousands of other people to reach the cupcake stall, you'll know for certain that you're not alone!

RECOMMENDED READING AND VIEWING

There are some amazing books and films out there that will inspire and inform. These are a few of our favourites!

Books

- ***Eating Animals***, by Jonathan Safran Foer: this book changes lives! 'Gripping, horrible, wonderful, breath-taking, original. A brilliant synthesis of argument, science and storytelling. One of the finest books ever written on the subject of eating animals,' says *The Times Literary Supplement*

- ***Why We Love Dogs, Eat Pigs and Wear Cows***, by Melanie Joy: an introduction by this vegan social psychologist author to 'carnism' – the ideology that conditions people to see some animals as food and others as friends. A powerful, fascinating book

- ***How Not to Die***, by Dr Michael Greger: scientifically proven nutritional advice on how to prevent our biggest killers – heart disease, breast and prostate cancers, diabetes and more

- ***Farmageddon: The True Cost of Cheap Meat***, by Philip Lymbery: what factory farming really means for animals, the planet and many of the world's poorest. An engaging read that packs a punch

- ***Esther the Wonder Pig***, by Steve Jenkins and Derek Walter: a wonderfully funny, inspiring story of how Esther, a 'micropig', changed the lives and perceptions of the people who adopted her

Films

- ***Cowspiracy***: follow the journey of film-maker Kip Andersen as he goes on a mission to uncover the environmental impact of our food choices. Engaging and compelling

- ***Vegucated***: three meat- and cheese-loving New Yorkers are challenged to go vegan for six weeks. Follow their highs and lows!

- ***Earthlings***: one of the most impactful films you will see. It's a tough watch, but one that will change how you view society's use of animals. Definitely not suitable for children

- ***Carnage***: comedian Simon Amstell's mockumentary, set in 2067, looking back to the bad old days when people actually ate animals. It's *very* funny!

- ***Forks Over Knives***: this thought-provoking, life-changing film presents the case for eating plant-based foods for our health. Always a popular choice with Veganuary participants

INFORMATION AND PRACTICAL SUPPORT

Got a question that isn't answered here? Or looking for further practical help? Veganuary.com has all the info you might need, as well as hundreds of tasty recipes.

WHAT HAPPENS ON DAY 32?

Some people try a month of plant-based eating, intending to be fully vegan by the end. Others are surprised that the 31-day challenge that had once seemed so daunting has become a way of life so quickly. Some people take part in Veganuary more than once, and enjoy each month of plant-based eating. Others, who have taken part several times, later come to decide they will remain a full-time vegan. Of those who try it but don't stay vegan, almost everyone still decides to reduce their consumption of animal products.

Whatever happens, happens. All we ask is that you give it your best shot for 31 days. Only when you break some of those old habits, form some new ones, try the many different products available and see how your body reacts to a fully plant-based diet – only then will you know whether you will want to stay vegan.

First and foremost, we want you to *try* vegan, but you won't be surprised to learn that we'd love you to *stay* vegan, too. That choice is yours alone, but for now, throw yourself into it. Embrace the challenge. Learn some new recipes. Make some new friends. See how your body feels. Discover what other changes it brings into your life. Be open-minded.

And on day 32 you will wake up, and you'll know what to do.

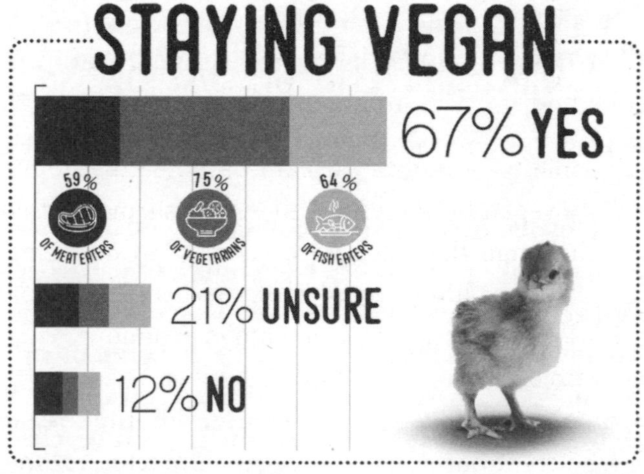

The survey results from Veganuary's #Classof2017 suggest most people commit to staying vegan after their one month pledge.

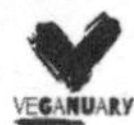

I THINK I'VE GONE VEGAN . . . WHAT NOW?

Not everyone expects to become vegan at the end of the 31 days but there are thousands who surprise themselves and take to veganism like a rescued factory-farmed duck to water. For them, this is just the beginning of a lifelong adventure, and they're hungry for more.

For those who love the social side, there are countless online vegan groups to check out. And in the real world, meet-up groups allow vegans to enjoy a meal together. Vegan festivals take place in towns and cities all over the world, and are always upbeat, rewarding events. At them, you'll meet like-minded people, discover great food, hear inspiring speakers and learn more about related campaigns. Maybe you'll even become an activist. You'll certainly eat a lot of cake.

If any of the issues touch your heart, you may feel empowered to make a difference by joining campaigns. It's not all banners and shouting. Lots of people give talks and cookery demonstrations in schools, or sign petitions, or share videos online, or make their own films. People write blogs, create websites and launch their own YouTube channels. Some write to newspapers, or hold a vegan coffee morning for charity.

Those who love sport may join a Vegan Runners or other athletes' group, or take inspiration from PlantBuilt or any number of extraordinary vegan athletes out there. There are lot of ways to be an ambassador for a vegan lifestyle, not least wearing the compassionate message emblazoned across your Lycra as you knock out a plant-based PB.

Perhaps you'll invite friends to a vegan meal to showcase how delicious the food can be, or take cakes or cookies into work along with the recipes, for those who'd like to make them at home. Maybe you'll visit the restaurants in your town and encourage them to offer a wider range of plant-based meals.

You might like to volunteer at your local animal sanctuary or take in some rescued hens. Or you may feel, as many new vegans do, a greater connection with nature, and you'll want to spend more time outdoors, watching the sun rise or listening to birdsong.

If you found this book helpful, maybe you'll buy more copies of it for friends and family. You may like to support Veganuary and help us make more vegans.

Or maybe you'll continue your life exactly as you did before, only you won't be eating animals.

Only you will know where veganism will take you.

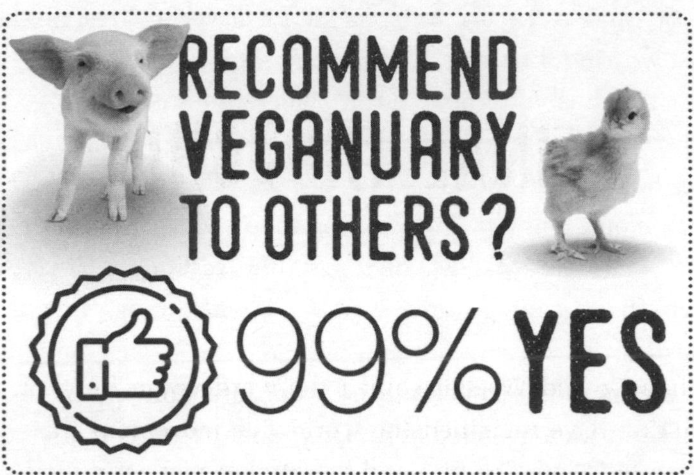

The survey results from Veganuary's #Classof2017 suggest almost all participants would recommend Veganuary to their friends.

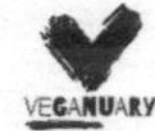

'This was the best decision of my life. I know lots of people say it, and I certainly mean it: I wish that I had been a vegan all of my life. The only regret I have about being a vegan is that I wish I'd done it sooner.'

Peter Egan, actor, UK,
Veganuary Class of 2016

FINAL THOUGHTS

When Donald Watson coined the word *vegan* in 1944, he couldn't have imagined the worldwide movement that was going to follow. For him and his band of pioneering friends, veganism was all about ending exploitation of animals. It was then, as it is now, a social justice movement. For many vegans, speciesism sits alongside racism and sexism as one more form of discrimination. After all, aren't we all just animals trying to do the best we can on this small planet we share?

Those early vegans wouldn't have known about the environmental devastation that animal agriculture would come to cause, or that people would starve while grain that could have sustained them was fed to farmed animals. Perhaps they wouldn't have known about the health benefits of a plant-based diet, either.

Today, we know a lot more. And the more we know, the more reasons we find to follow their lead.

Being vegan spares the suffering of animals that most of us cannot bear even to watch. It reduces our impact on the planet and safeguards it for the future. And it protects our health against some of the most common causes of death: heart disease, stroke, diabetes and some cancers.

Thank you for thinking more carefully about your food choices, for pledging to try veganism for a month, for one day a week or for the rest of your life. Every vegan meal we eat makes a difference. Each one is an affirmation that we want a kinder, fairer and healthier world, and that we won't wait for someone else to create it.

Those 31 days may well change your life, and if you decide once the month is over that staying vegan is the right choice for you, well, Veganuary will be on hand to advise, mentor and support you should you need it. Get in touch anyway. We'd love to hear from you.

MORE ON VEGANUARY

Visit veganuary.com for more information on animals, the environment, nutrition, health, eating out, accidentally vegan products, shopping, recommended reading and viewing and hundreds of delicious plant-based recipes.

Veganuary (pronounced vee-gan-uary) is a UK charity with international reach that encourages people to try vegan in January (or any time of year), and offers support and advice for the process. Tens of thousands of people from more than 100 countries have already taken part.

Most people who sign up for the month are meat-eaters or pescatarians (people who eat fish but no other meat), but many are vegetarians, too. Whatever your diet, wherever you're from and whatever your age or gender, all are welcome.

It's totally free to take part in Veganuary, and everyone who signs up receives:

- Daily emails with shopping lists, eating-out guides, nutrition advice, recipes, meal plans and answers to common questions

- Social media support in our closed Facebook group. Here you can connect with other participants from around the world, and share your experiences

- A free celebrity e-cookbook, with delicious animal-free recipes

- Competitions with great prizes to be won, and special offers from some of your favourite companies

- Someone available throughout the month to answer any questions you may have

We aim to make the month enjoyable and interesting. We encourage and support; we never judge. Around two-thirds of those who take part in Veganuary enjoy it so much that they choose to stay vegan at the end of the month, and almost everyone else chooses to become vegetarian or reduce their consumption of animal products. Some people take part in Veganuary every year; others take part for several years before deciding to become vegan. Which path you choose is up to you.

'Thanks to this group and its awesome support and positivity, I am so proud that I not only smashed January but have continued into March without a hiccup. This is a life choice for me now . . . one I actually always wanted to make but for some reason doubted I could do . . . so I just wanted to say *Thank you.'*

Vickie D., Millswood, South Australia,
Veganuary Class of 2017

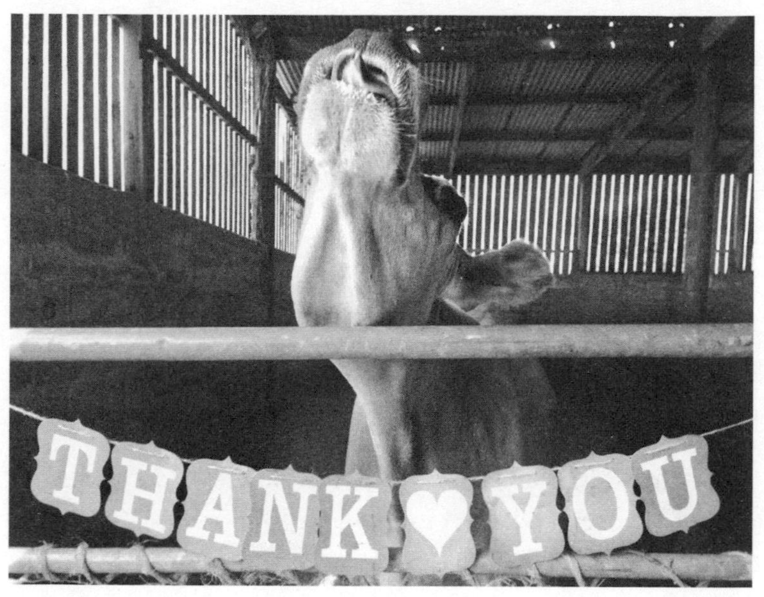
THANK ♥ YOU

ABOUT THE AUTHOR

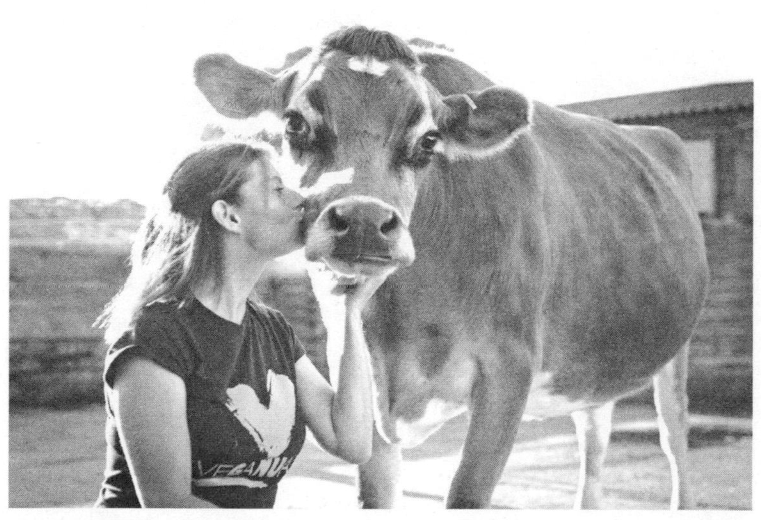

Kate Schuler became vegan in 1992 after the shock of discovering that cows and chickens were killed in the dairy and egg industries as well as for meat. After her first seven days as a vegan, her resolve temporarily failed and she gorged on cheese. Afterwards, when feeling sick with guilt and sick with cheese, she vowed never to eat animal products again. Since then, she has worked with more than a dozen pro-vegan organisations and businesses to make the case for a plant-based world. One mark of progress is that there are now ten vegan cheeses for sale within a mile of her home. Kate lives in Sussex, UK and shares her home with rescued dogs, rabbits and a cat named Jess, to whom she and her partner Christopher have pledged their devoted servitude.

NOTES

Introduction

1 'Top Trends in Prepared Foods 2017: Exploring trends in meat, fish and seafood; pasta, noodles and rice; prepared meals; savory deli food; soup; and meat substitutes', Global Data website, June 2017
2 'Vegan Society Poll', Ipsos Mori website, 17 May 2016
3 'KaTech targets fast-growing vegan trends', Food Ingredients First website, 30 Aug 2017
4 'More tofu? Supermarkets flesh out their vegan credentials as clean eating grows', Sarah Butler, *Guardian*, 27 May 2017
5 'Australia is the third-fastest growing vegan market in the world', Lucy Cormack, *The Sydney Morning Herald*, 5 Jun 2016

For Animals

1 'Do people know where their chicken comes from?', Tom de Castella, BBC News website, 23 Oct 2014

2 'Farm animals need our help', American Society for the Prevention of Cruelty to Animals website
3 'The Case Against Cages: Evidence in favour of alternative systems for laying hens,' RSPCA website
4 'USDA weekly egg price and inventory report', Egg News, 20 Sept 2017
5 'Unscrambled: the hidden truth of hen welfare in the Australian egg industry', Voiceless website, May 2017
6 'At slaughter', Animal Welfare Institute website
7 'Dairy cows fact sheet', Animals Australia website
8 '"A national disgrace": Catalogue of suffering at Scottish abattoirs revealed', Bureau of Investigative Journalism website, 19 Apr 2017
9 'Maternal slaughter at abattoirs: history, causes, cases and the meat industry', *Springer Plus*, 22 Mar 2013
10 'Pregnant cows face slaughter as milk contracts not renewed', Brad Thompson Harvey, *The West Australian*, 1 Oct 2016
11 'Slaughter of pregnant cattle in German abattoirs - current situation and prevalence: a cross-sectional study', *BMC Veterinary Research*, 7 Jun 2016
12 Singleton, G.H. and Dobson, H. 'A survey of the reasons for culling pregnant cows', *Veterinary Record 136*, 1995
13 'Grazing-based dairying: How the U.S. compares to other countries', Peter van Elzakker, *Progressive Dairyman*, 20 Sept 2013
14 'Pain management issues when castrating and dehorning', Heather Smith Thomas, *Progressive Cattleman*, 25 June 2015

15 'Restaurants drive up cattle slaughter age in quest for more mature beef flavour', Laura Poole, ANB News website, 16 Jul 2015

16 'How do Canada's welfare standards compete worldwide?', Jennifer Jackson, Farms website, 9 May 2017

17 'Why is nest-building behaviour so important?', FreeFarrowing website

18 'Guidance: caring for pigs', Department for Environment, Food & Rural Affairs, UK Government website, 8 Apr 2013

19 D. M. Weary and D. Fraser, 'Calling by domestic piglets: reliable signals of need?', *Animal Behaviour*, 1995; 50(4), 1047–1055

20 'The life of – Pigs', Compassion in World Farming website, 20 May 2013

21 Ibid.

22 'Handy hints: three ways to manipulate a sheep's breeding cycle', Louise Hartley, *Farmers Guardian*, 8 Oct 2014

23 'End to the silence about 15 million dead lambs', Sue Neales, *The Australian*, 3 Sept 2012

24 'Lambing Part 4 – ensuring survival of newborn lambs', National Animal Disease Information Service website

25 'Managing newborn lambs', Volac International Limited

26 'Handy hints: three ways to manipulate a sheep's breeding cycle', Louise Hartley, *Farmers Guardian*, 8 Oct 2014

27 'Guidelines on the examination of rams for breeding', Sheep Veterinary Society website, June 2014

28 'Artificial insemination in sheep', Paula I. Menzies, Ontario Veterinary College, University of Guelph, published by Merck & Co

29 'Up to 70 sheep drown in "freak" flash flooding near Llanrwst', Tom Davidson, *Daily Post*, 11 Dec 2015
30 'Sheep guide: a guide to fly strike', That's Farming website, 31 May 2017
31 'Farmers call for help over mounting sheep deaths', Sarah Butler, *Guardian*, 3 Apr 2013
32 'Lamb', glossary, BBC Good Food website
33 'Managing cull ewes', Agriculture and Horticulture Development Board website, 31 Aug 2016
34 'Unilateral eyestalk ablation', Laboratory of Aquaculture and Artemia Reference Center, Ghent University
35 'Why we need bees: nature's tiny workers put food on our tables', National Resources Defense Council website, Mar 2011
36 Wheeler, M.M., Robinson, G.E. 'Diet-dependent gene expression in honey bees: Honey vs sucrose or high fructose corn syrup'. *Scientific Reports* 4, Article number: 5726 (2014)

For the Environment

1 '10 ways vegetarianism can help save the planet', John Vidal, *Guardian*, 18 Jul 2010
2 'The impact of animal farming on people and planet', Quaker Council for European Affairs website
3 G. Myhre., et al. 'Anthropogenic and natural radiative forcing', *Climate Change 2013: The Physical Science Basis.*

Contribution of working group / report of the Intergovernmental Panel on Climate Change, 2013

4 'Greenhouse gas emissions', United States Environmental Protection Agency website

5 'Do the UN's new numbers for livestock emissions kill the argument for vegetarianism?', Emma Bryce, *Guardian*, 27 Sept 2013

6 Wynes, S. and Nicholas, K.A., 'The climate mitigation gap: education and government recommendations miss the most effective individual actions', Environmental Research Letters, Volume 12, Number 7, 12 Jul 2017

7 'Water scarcity: overview', World Wildlife Fund For Nature website

8 'The looming threat of water scarcity', Worldwatch Institute website, 19 Mar 2013

9 Ibid.

10 '10 ways vegetarianism can help save the planet', John Vidal, *Guardian*, 18 Jul 2010

11 Ibid.

12 Ibid.

13 'Water-poor Saudi Arabia moves farming venture to drought-stricken California', Matt Weiser, *Guardian*, 8 Mar 2016

14 '10 ways vegetarianism can help save the planet', John Vidal, *Guardian*, 18 Jul 2010

15 'Water requirements', Vegan Society website

16 'Cost effective slurry storage strategies on dairy farms', DairyCo, AHDB Dairy website, Feb 2010

17 'Number of cattle worldwide from 2012 to 2017 (in million head)', Statista website, 2017
18 'Pollution from industrialised livestock production', Food and Agriculture Organization website
19 'Toothless Environment Agency is allowing the living world to be wrecked with impunity', George Monbiot, *Guardian,* 12 Nov 2015
20 '10 ways vegetarianism can help save the planet', John Vidal, *Guardian,* 18 Jul 2010
21 Ibid.
22 'Environmental and health problems in livestock production: pollution in the food system', The Agribusiness Accountability Initiative
23 'Farming "hotspots" carry air pollution risk, Dutch study finds', Pilita Clark, *Financial Times,* 2 Sep 2016
24 Alavanja, M.C.R., 'Pesticides Use and Exposure Extensive Worldwide', *Reviews on Environmental Health.* 2009;24(4): 303-309
25 'Shocking declines in bird numbers show British wildlife is "in serious trouble"', Ian Johnston, *Independent,* 19 May 2017
26 '"Dramatic" decline in European birds linked to industrial agriculture', *Deutsche Welle,* 4 May 2017
27 'The State of Canada's birds 2012', North American Bird Conservation Initiative, Canada, May 2012
28 'Fact check: does Australia have one of the "highest loss of species anywhere in the world?"' ABC News website
29 'Land cover change in Queensland 2014–15', Queensland Government, 2016, p.21

30 "Tree-clearing causing Queensland's greatest animal welfare crisis', World Wildlife Fund for Nature website, 6 Sept 2017

31 'State of Nature 2016', State of Nature Partnership

32 'Agriculture and overuse greater threats to wildlife than climate change – study', Jessica Aldred, *Guardian*, 10 Aug 2016

33 Ibid.

34 'Forest conversion', World Wildlife Fund for Nature website

35 'Amazon deforestation report is major setback for Brazil ahead of climate talks', Jonathan Watts, *Guardian*, 27 Nov 2015

36 'Most of Amazon rainforest's species extinctions are yet to come', Helen Thompson, *Scientific American*, 13 Jul 2012

37 'The Sumatran rainforest will mostly disappear within 20 years', John Vidal, *Observer*, 26 May 2013

38 Philip Lymbery, *Dead Zone: Where the Wild Things Were*, Bloomsbury, 2017

39 'The oilpalm connection: is the Sumatran elephant the price of our cheap meat?', Philip Lymbery, *The Ecologist*, 28 Mar 2017

40 'Deforestation and climate change', Greenpeace website

41 'Monsters of the oceans: 7 criminal super trawlers that threaten our waters', Greenpeace Australia Pacific, 19 Nov 2014

42 'The boy who stole Queen Victoria's knickers, and 19 other fascinating facts about Buckingham Palace,' Soo Kim, *The Telegraph*, 7 Apr 2017

43 '5 reasons you should be worried about super trawlers', Animals Australia website, 20 Sept 2017

44 Ibid.

45 'Overfishing', World Wildlife Fund for Nature website
46 'Ocean fish stocks on "verge of collapse" says IRIN report', Azua (Zizhan) Luo, *NewsecurityBeat*, 28 Feb 2017
47 'New US regulations offer better protection from bycatch', *World Wildlife Fund Magazine*, Spring 2017
48 'Māui dolphin', World Wildlife Fund for Nature website
49 'Reducing bycatch of North Atlantic right whales', World Wildlife Fund for Nature website
50 'Bycatch – wasteful and destructive fishing', Greenpeace
51 'Terrible toll of fishing nets on seabirds revealed', Daniel Cressey, *Nature*, 29 May 2013
52 'Impacts of the Peruvian anchoveta supply chains: from wild fish in the water to protein on the plate', *Globec International Newsletter*, Apr 2010
53 'Overfishing and El Niño push the world's biggest single-species fishery to a critical point', Allison Guy, Oceana website, 2 Feb 2016

Sustainability and World Hunger

1 'We already grow enough food for 10 billion people – and still can't end hunger', Eric Holtz Gimenez, *Huffington Post*, 2 May 2012
2 'Food', United Nations website
3 Global warning: the impact of meat production and consumption on climate change. Pachauri, R. Compassion in World Farming. 8 Sept, 2008

4 '10 ways vegetarianism can help save the planet', John Vidal, *Guardian*, 18 Jul 2010

5 Ibid.

6 'A five-step plan to feed the world' Jonathan Foley, *National Geographic Magazine*, May 2014

7 'World Livestock 2011: Livestock in food security', Food and Agriculture Organization of the United Nations, 2011, p. 21

8 'Livestock – Climate change's forgotten sector: global public opinion on meat and dairy consumption', R. Bailey et al., Chatham House, 3 Dec 2014, p. 13

For Personal Health

1 'The top 10 causes of death', World Health Organization website, Jan 2017

2 Bradbury K.E. et al, 'Serum concentrations of cholesterol, apolipoprotein A-I and apolipoprotein B in a total of 1694 meat-eaters, fish-eaters, vegetarians and vegans', *European Journal of Clinical Nutrition*, 2014 Feb; 68, 178–183 (February 2014)

3 'About cholesterol', American Heart Association website

4 'Fats explained', British Heart Foundation website

5 Alexander S. et al., 'A plant-based diet and hypertension. *Journal of Geriatric Cardiology*, 2017; 14(5), 327–330

6 'Obesity Statistics, Briefing Paper', Carl Baker, House of Commons Library, 20 Jan 2017

7 Tonstad S., et al., 'Type of Vegetarian Diet, Body Weight, and

Prevalence of Type 2 Diabetes'. *Diabetes Care*. 2009;32(5), 791–796

8 Tuso P.J., et al., 'Nutritional Update for Physicians: Plant-Based Diets'. *The Permanente Journal*. 2013;17(2),61–66

9 'Obesity? Diabetes? We've been set up,' Alvin Powell, *Harvard Gazette*, 7 Mar 2012

10 Michael Greger, *How Not To Die*, Flatiron Books, 2015, p. 106

11 'Diabetes in Australia', Diabetes Australia website

12 'Twenty devastating amputations every day', Diabetes UK website, 30 Aug 2016

13 Lee. Y., Park, K. 'Adherence to a vegetarian diet and diabetes risk: a systematic review and meta-analysis of observational studies.' *Nutrients* 2017, 9(6), 603

14 Ibid.

15 'Type 2 diabetes can be reversed in just four months, trial shows', Sarah Knapton, *Telegraph*, 15 Mar 2017

16 'Vegetarian diets and diabetes', Diabetes UK website

17 'Q&A on the carcinogenicity of the consumption of red meat and processed meat', World Health Organization, Oct 2015

18 Ibid

19 'Processed meats do cause cancer - WHO', James Gallagher, BBC News website, 26 Oct 2015

20 'Bacon and sausages sales down after cancer scare report', Lexi Finnigan, *Telegraph*, 22 Nov 2015

21 Kizil, M., et al. 'A review on the formation of carcinogenic/mutagenic heterocyclic aromatic amines. *Journal of Food Processing and Technology*, 2:5 (2011)

22 Zheng, W., Lee, S.A. 'Well-done Meat Intake, Heterocyclic Amine Exposure, and Cancer Risk'. *Nutrition and Cancer.* 2009;61(4):437–446

23 'Foodborne illnesses', National Institute of Diabetes and Digestive and Kidney Diseases website

24 'On call: diet, testicular cancer, and prostate cancer', Harvard Health Publishing website, Mar 2014

25 Melina, V., et. al., 'Position of the Academy of Nutrition and Dietetics: Vegetarian Diets.' *Journal of the Academy of Nutrition and Dietetics,* 2016 Dec;116(12):1970–1980

For Global Health

1 '10 things you didn't know about bird flu', Michael Greger, *The Ecologist,* 4 Feb 2009

2 'Farm animals consume nearly half of all antibiotics', Philip Lymbery, Compassion in World Farming website, 16 Nov 2011

3 'Deadly bird flu strains created by industrial poultry farms', Robert G. Wallace, *The Ecologist,* 30 Jan 2017

4 'UK on track to cut antibiotic use in animals as total sales drop 9%', Department for Environment, Food & Rural Affairs, UK Government website, 17 Nov 2016

5 'Antibiotics for animals to be restricted under government plans to beat drug resistance', Sarah Knapton, *Telegraph,* 13 May 2016

6 'Secrecy surrounding antibiotic use on Australian farms

sparks superbug fears', Melissa Davey, *Guardian*, 21 Sept 2016

7 'UK on track to cut antibiotic use in animals as total sales drop 9%', Department for Environment, Food & Rural Affairs, UK Government website, 17 Nov 2016

8 'Secrecy surrounding antibiotic use on Australian farms sparks superbug fears', Melissa Davey, *Guardian*, 21 Sept 2016

9 'Is it time for an antibiotic-free label on our food?', Tom Levitt, *Guardian*, 18 Jun 2015

For the Adventure

1 'A nation of aspiring foodies stuck in a nine-meal rut', Ocado Group website, 22 Feb 2015

Nutrition in a Nutshell

1 Nair, R., Maseeh, A. 'Vitamin D: The "sunshine" vitamin'. *Journal of Pharmacology & Pharmacotherapeutics*. 2012;3(2):118-126

2 'Vitamin D deficiency associated with heightened depression, study finds', Ian Johnston, *independent*, 19 Oct 2016

3 'Iron', National Health Service website

4 'Iron', National Institutes of Health website

5 'Food sources of iron', Dietitians of Canada, 18 Oct 2016

6 Michael Greger, *How Not To Die,* Flatiron Books, 8 Dec 2015, p.71
7 Etemadi, A., Mortality from different causes associated with meat, heme iron, nitrates, and nitrites in the NIH-AARP Diet and Health Study: population based cohort study. *BMJ 2017;357:j1957*
8 Zivkovic, A.M., et al., 'Dietary omega-3 fatty acids aid in the modulation of inflammation and metabolic health.' *California Agriculture.* 2011;65(3):106-111
9 'Ask the expert: omega-3 fatty acids', Harvard School of Public Health website, 19 June 2007
10 'The vegetarian diet', NHS website
11 'Meet Mungo', *The Washington Post,* 19 Apr 2003
12 'Everything you need to know about vitamin B12 deficiency', Nic Fleming, *Guardian,* 28 Feb 2017
13 'B vitamins and folic acid,' NHS website

Vegan Myths

1 '10 ways vegetarianism can help save the planet', John Vidal, *Guardian,* 18 Jul 2010
2 Scarborough, P., et al. Climatic Change (2014) 125: 179
3 Metges C.C., Barth C.A. 'Metabolic Consequences of a High Dietary-Protein Intake in Adulthood: Assessment of the Available Evidence.' *Journal of Nutrition April 1, 2000 vol. 130 no. 4 886-889*

4 'The protein myth: why you need less protein than you think', Jessica Jones, *Huffington Post*, 21 Sept 2012

5 'Food fact sheet: vegetarian diets', British Dietetic Association website

6 'Lambing to order!', Tim Tyne, *Country Smallholding*, 6 May 2014

7 Song, M., et. al,. 'Association of Animal and Plant Protein Intake With All-Cause and Cause-Specific Mortality.' *JAMA Internal Medicine.* 2016;176(10):1453–1463

8 'Q&A on the carcinogenicity of the consumption of red meat and processed meat,' World Health Organization website, Oct 2015

9 'Processed meat and cancer – what you need to know', Cancer Research UK website, 26 Oct 2015

10 Ibid.

11 'Red meat and the risk of bowel cancer', NHS website

12 'Factors with less clear effect on prostate cancer risk', American Cancer Society website

13 'The five worst contaminants in chicken products', Physicians Committee for Responsible Medicine website

14 'Campylobacter', Food Standards Agency website

15 'Yearly food-borne illness estimates for Canada', Government of Canada website

16 '*Campylobacter* (Campylobacteriosis)', Centers for Disease Control and Prevention website

17 'Salmonella', Centers for Disease Control and Prevention website

18 'Almost $10 million for salmonella research', McGill University website, 21 Jul 2015

19 'Amazon rainforest's final frontier under threat from oil and soya', John Vidal, *Guardian*, 16 Feb 2017

20 'Soy is everywhere', World Wide Fund for Nature website

21 Ibid.

PICTURE ACKNOWLEDGEMENTS

Images pages vii, 19, 20, 129 (above and below), 167 © Chris Shoebridge Photography

Images pages 14, 17, 21 © Animal Equality

All other images © Veganuary